BARBER

We will cut just the way You want!

Give us a try

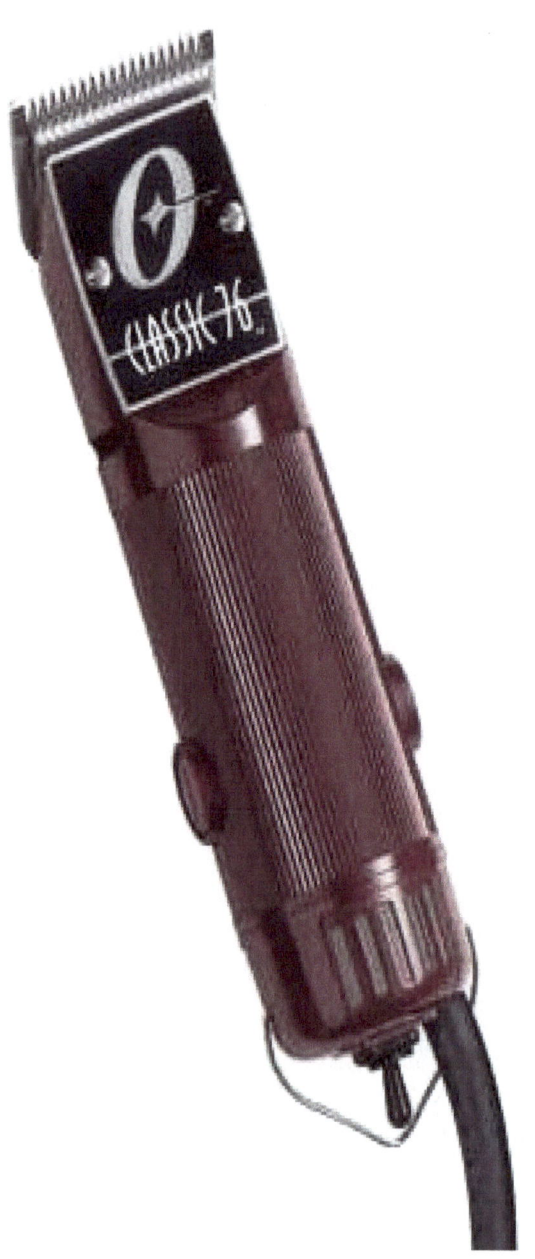

editor's note

Greetings,

    Welcome to another thrilling issue of The Barber Stylist Magazine. This issue is for the believers that know dreams do come true. Keep believing in yourself in all aspects of your life.

    The Barber Stylist Magazine is especially catered to the barbers and the stylists that know that satisfying their client is the first step in building longevity in the industry of grooming hair. The African American man and woman desire to look their best at all times. We are here as professionals to make sure that the clients feel and look the part for their careers, personal life, and all opportunities of life.

    The Barber Stylist Magazine is always dedicated to aspiring barbers and stylists that believe in their visions of tomorrow in the industry that they love the most. Take your time and build your marketing strategy and your talent to build your clientele for now and the future. Success is the key.

    The different hairstyles are here to help you grow and to better you craft. Remember to be yourself always.

Thanks So Much,

Dr. Roderick Van Daniel

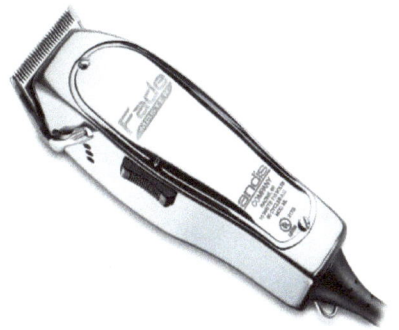

"The Barber Stylist Magazine"
(Semi-annual publication – Spring and Fall)

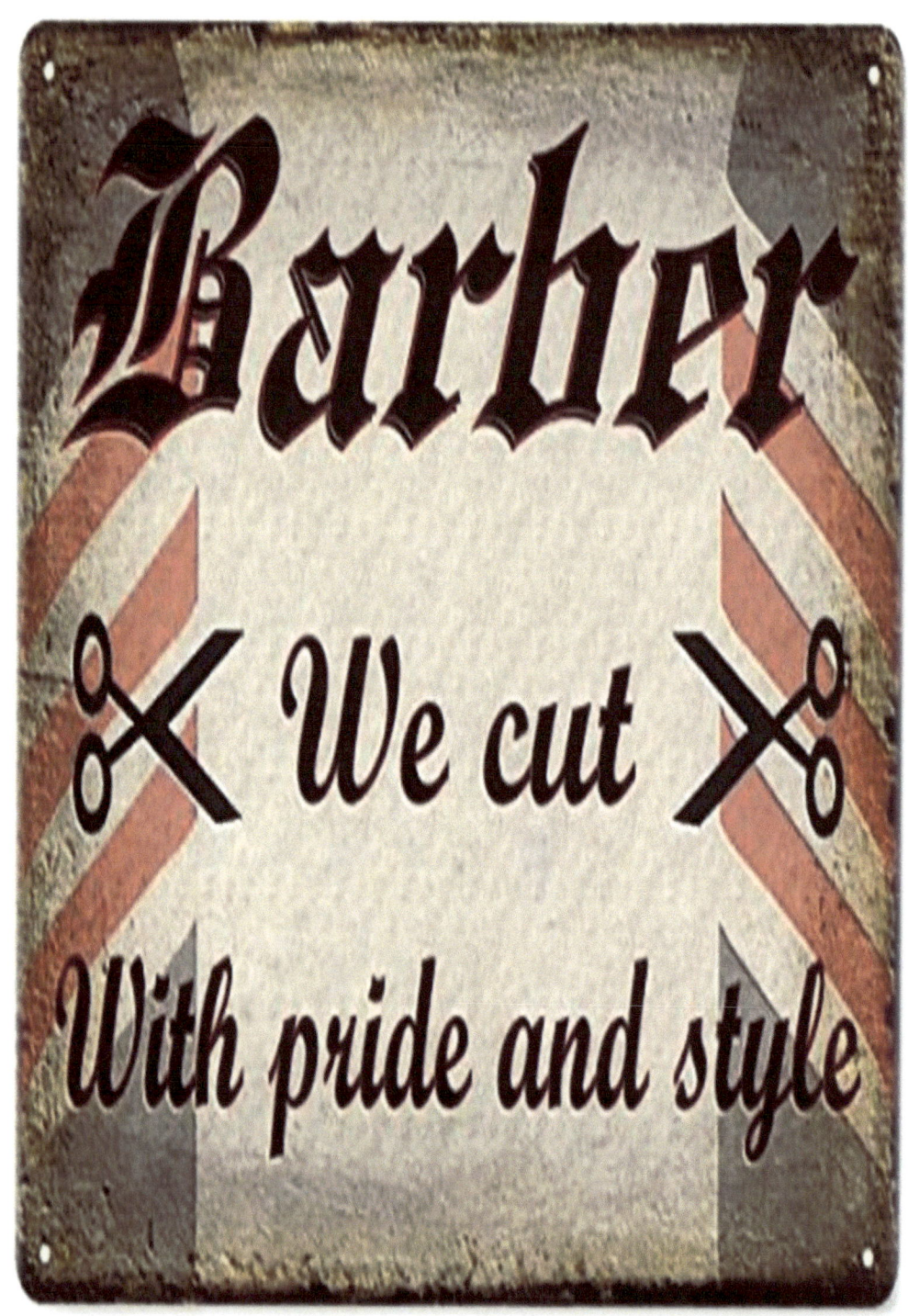

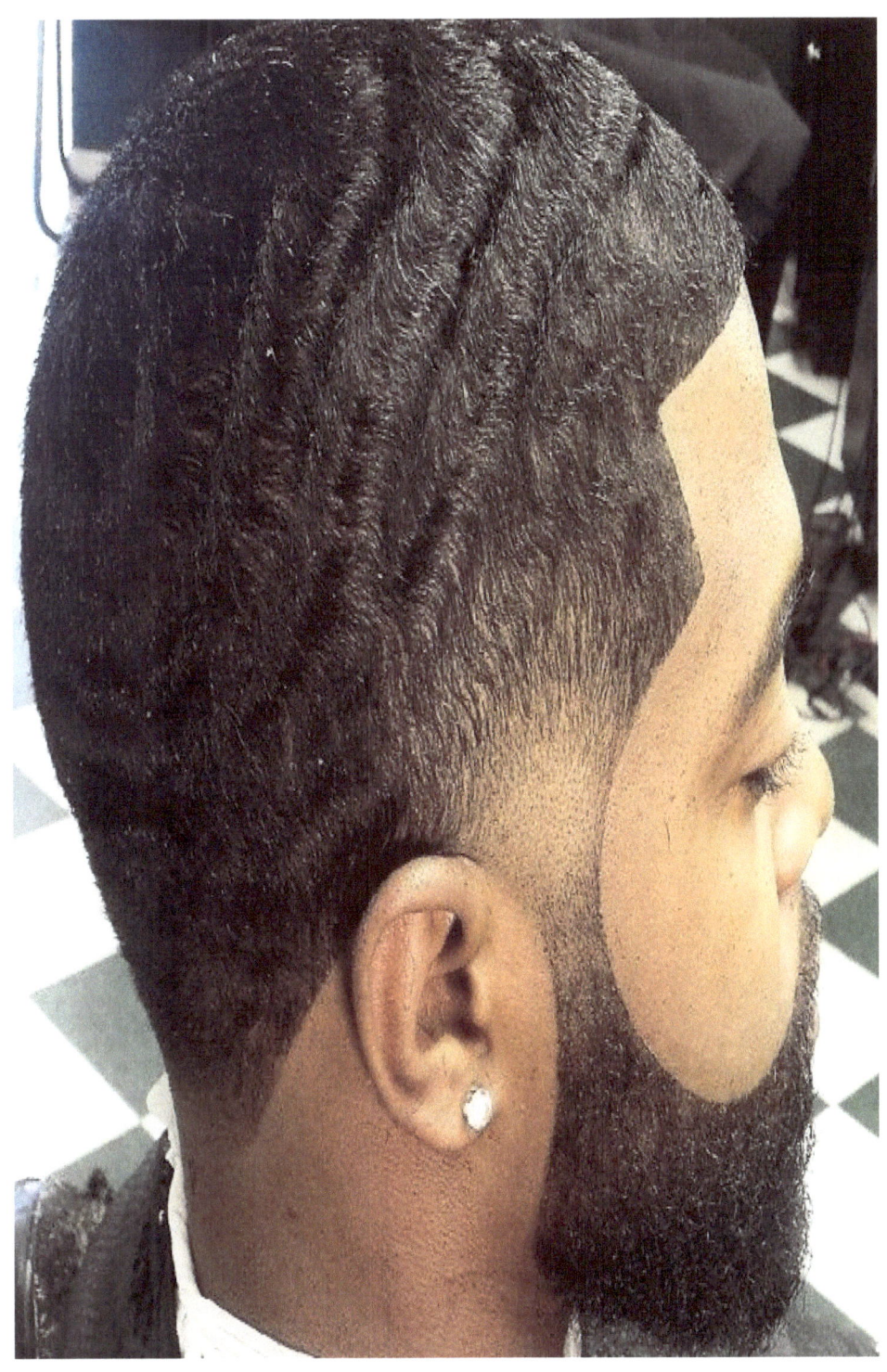

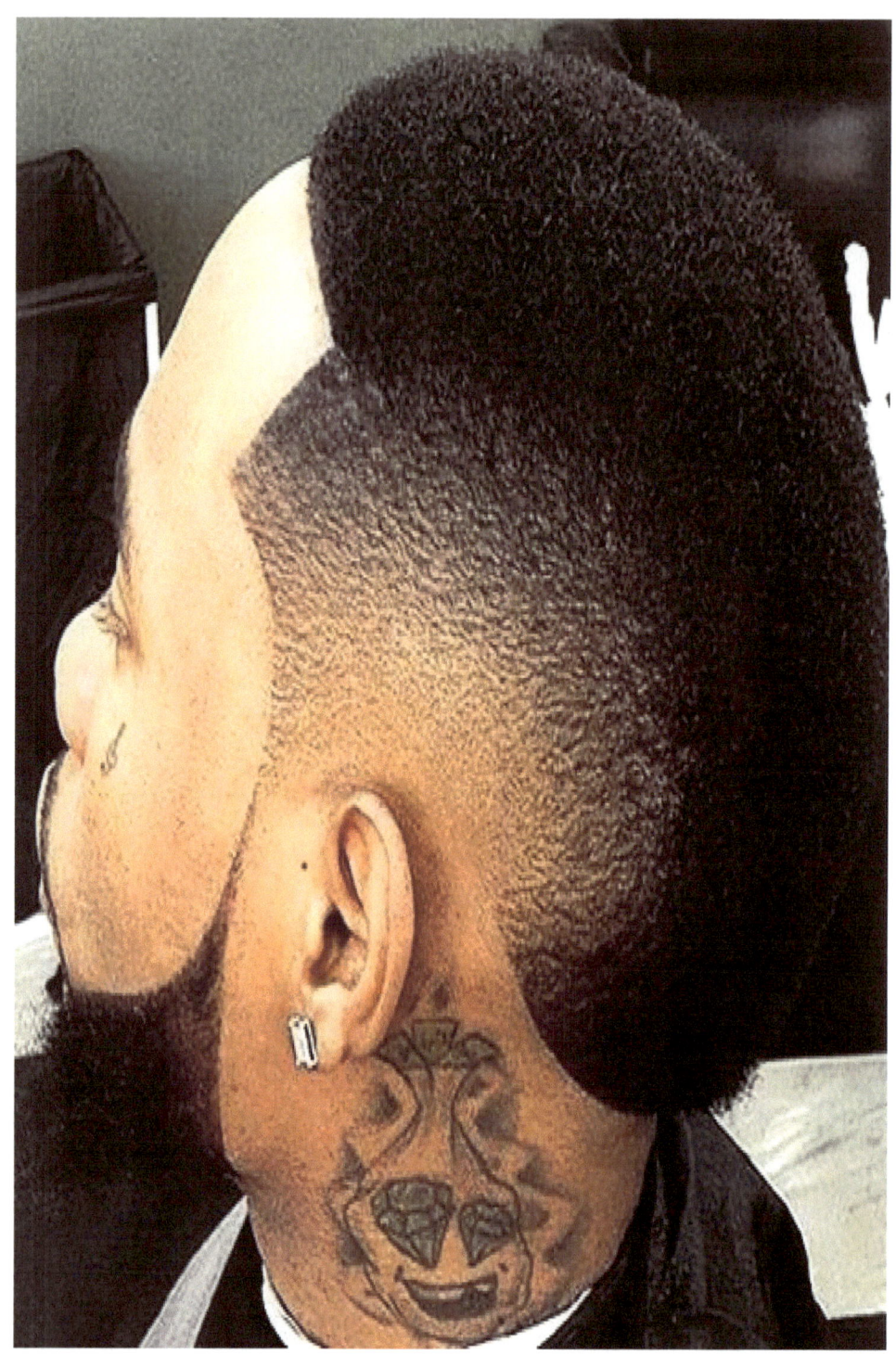

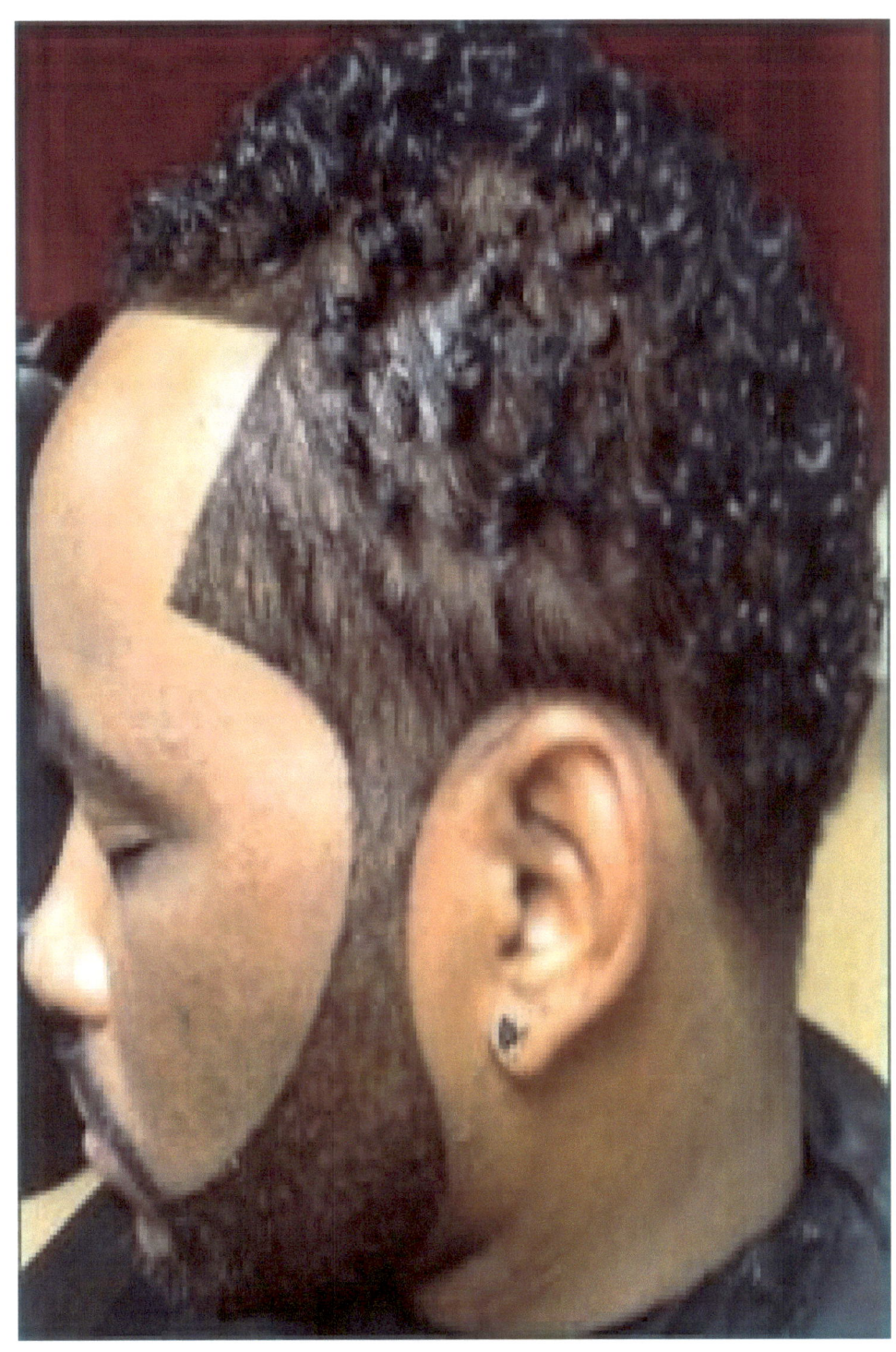

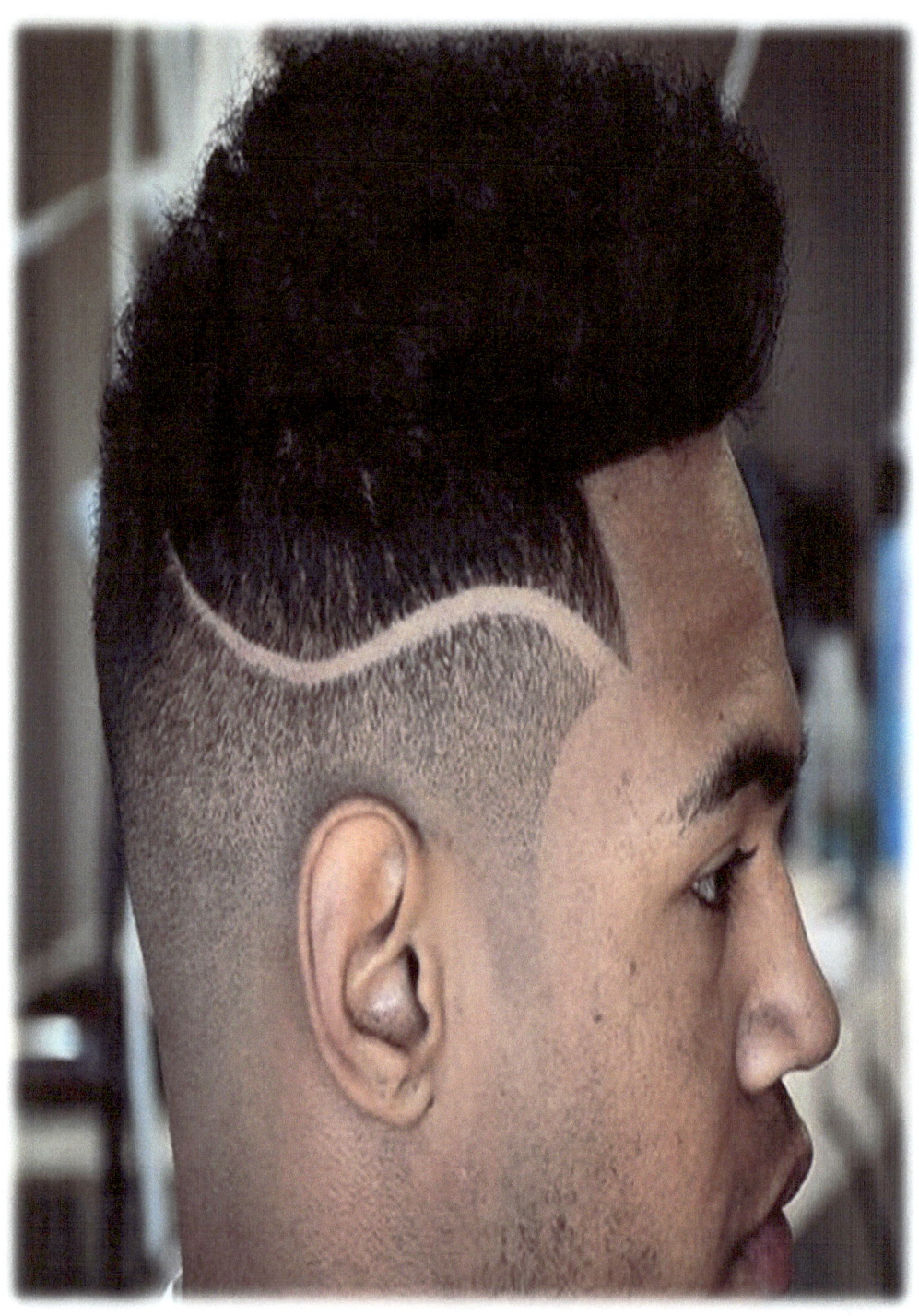

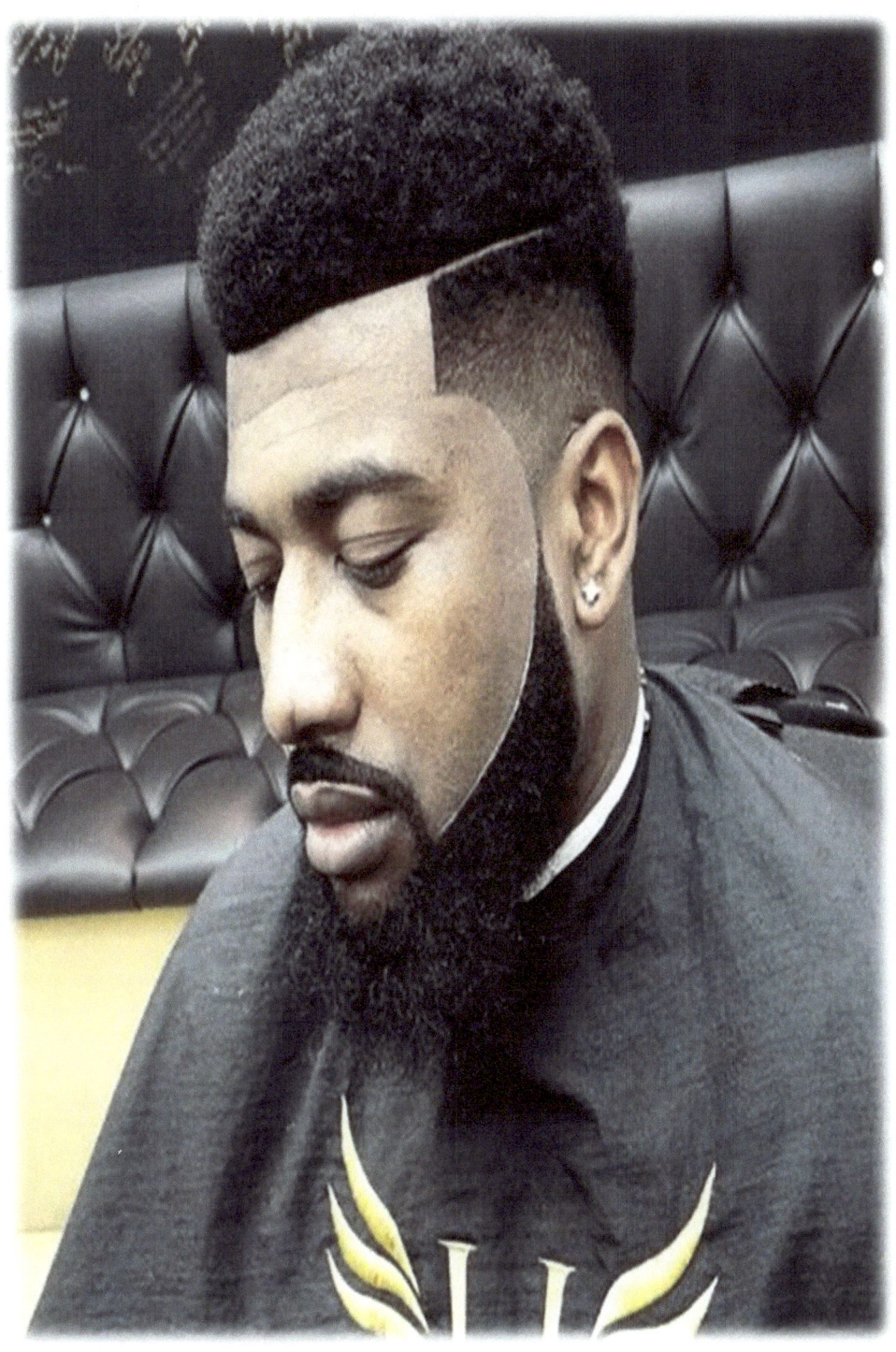

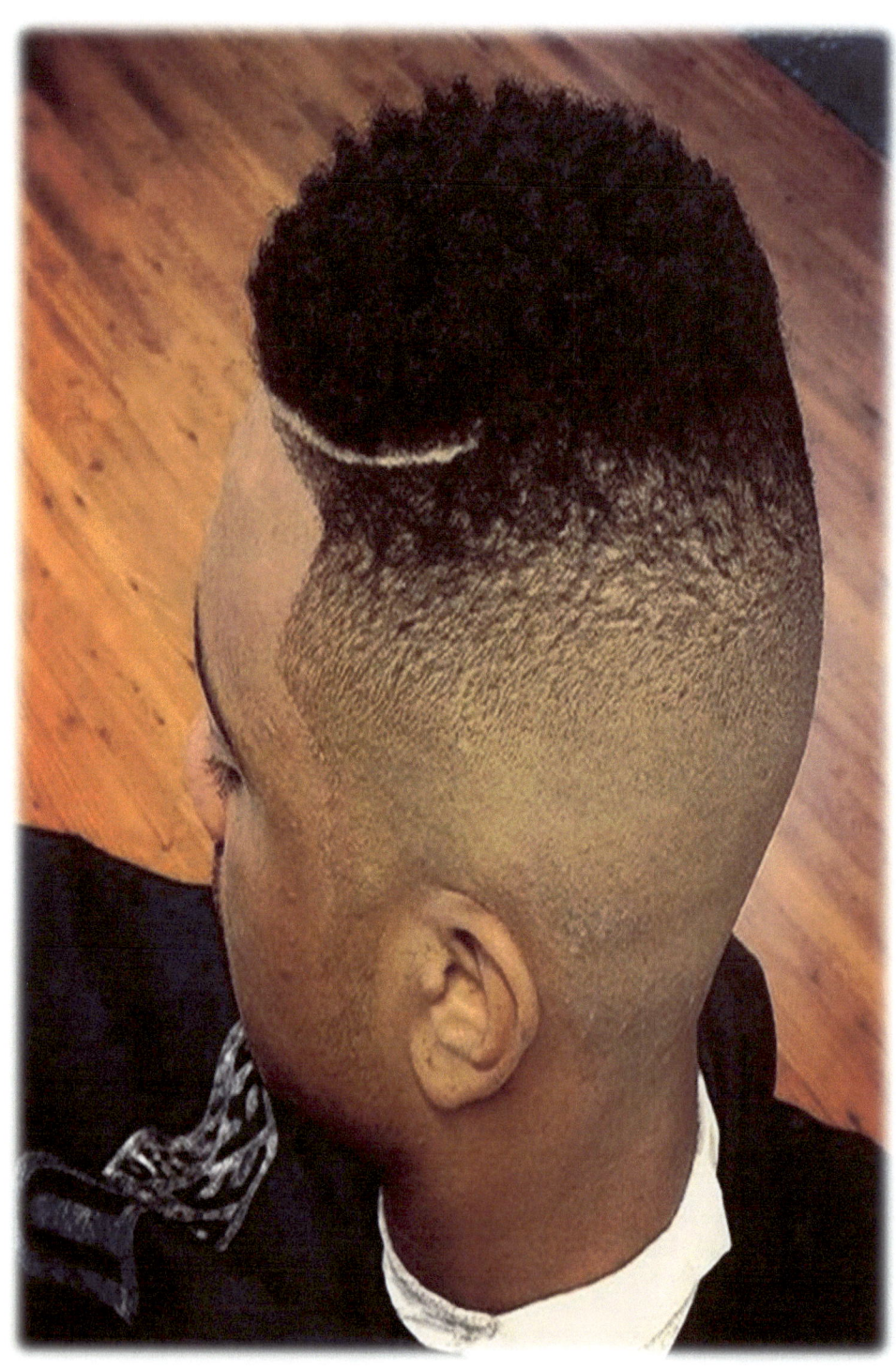

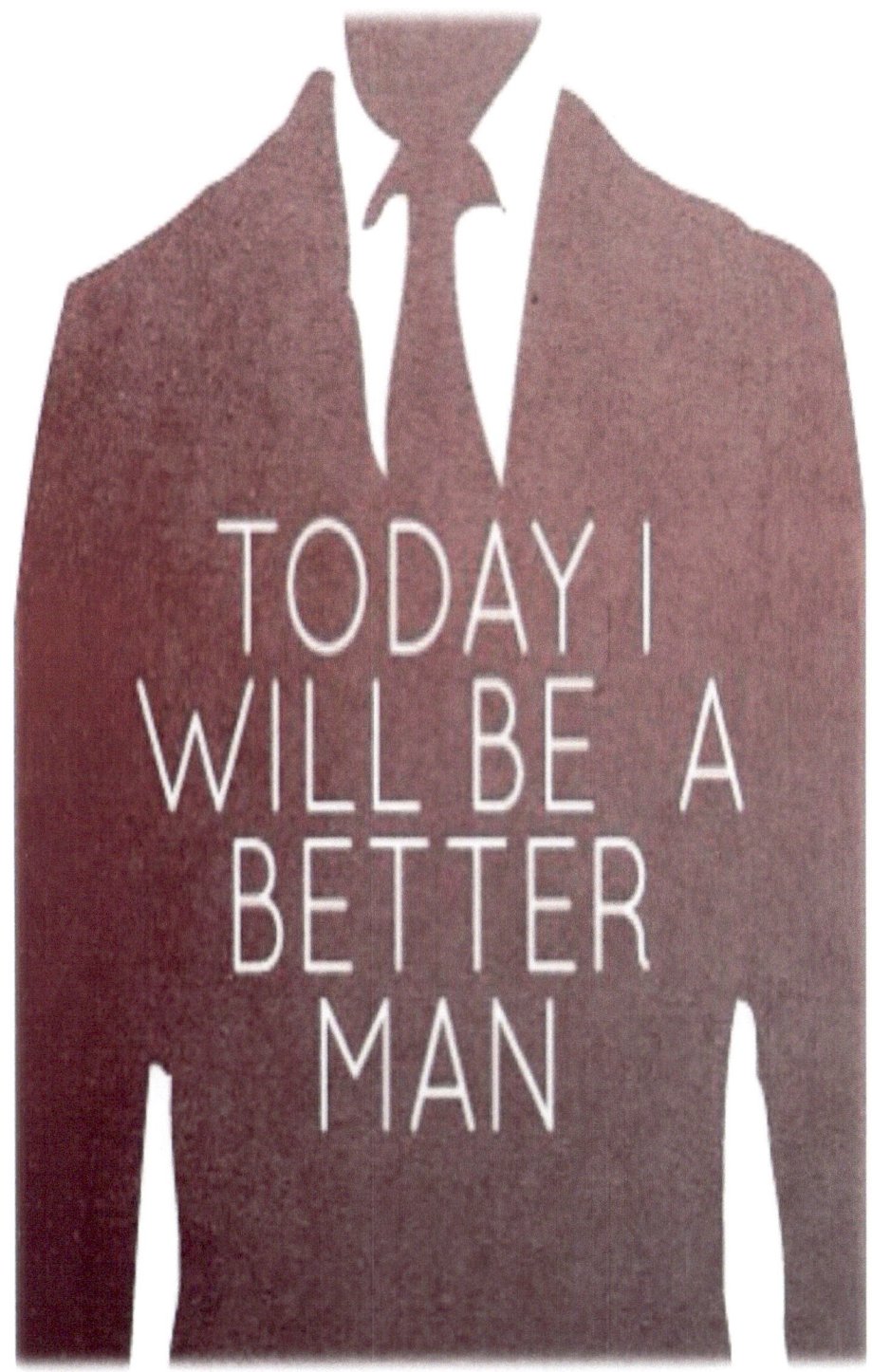

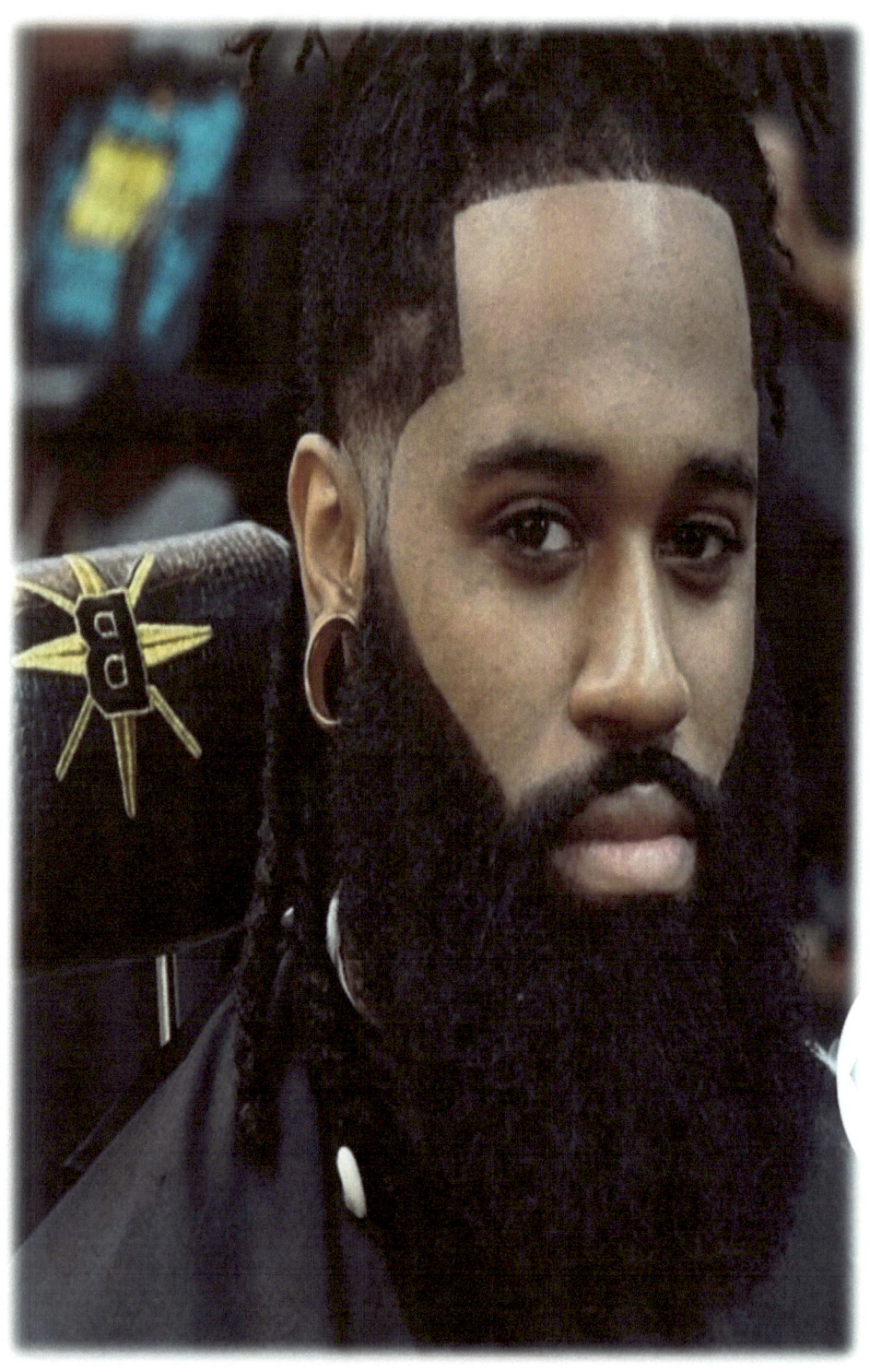

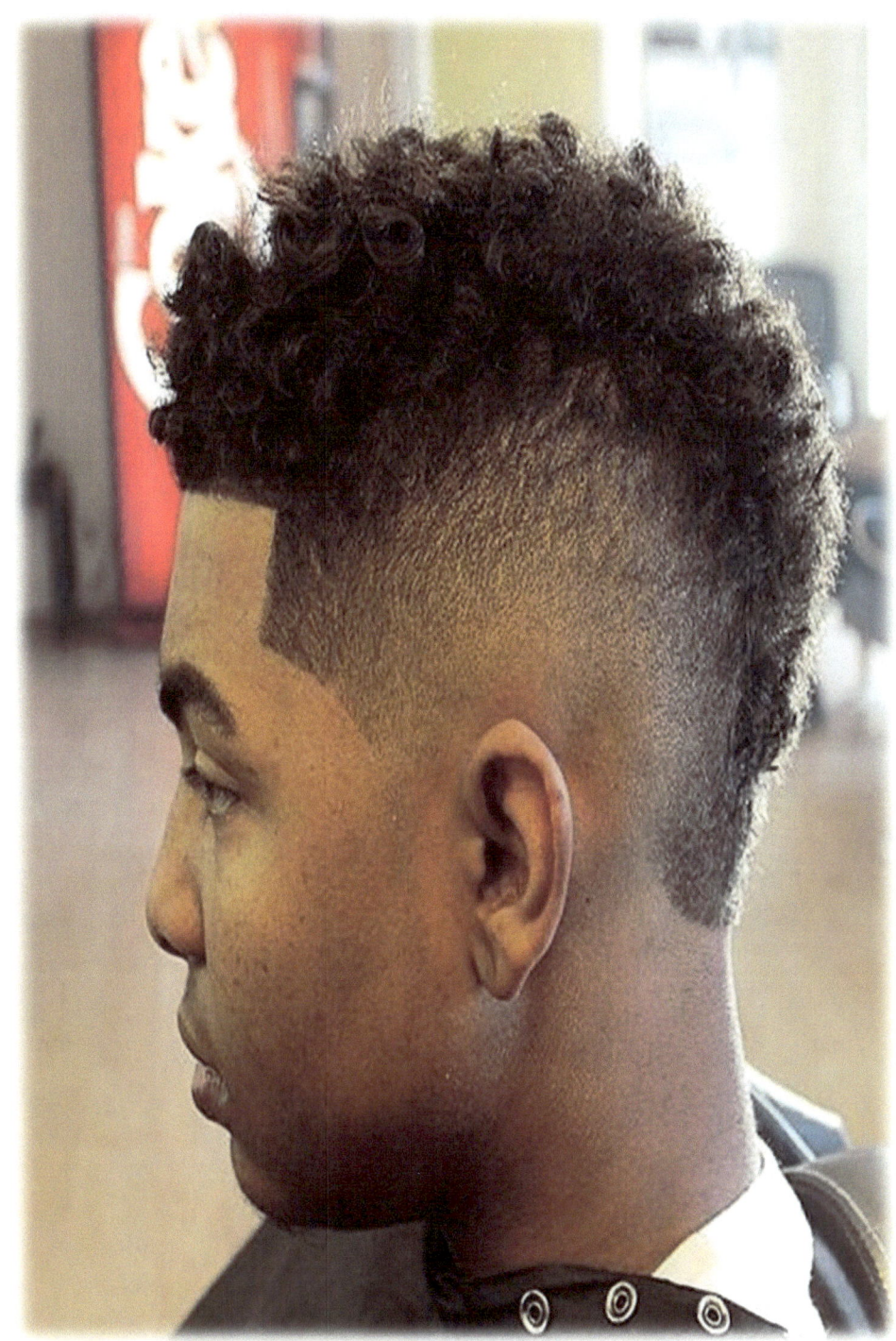

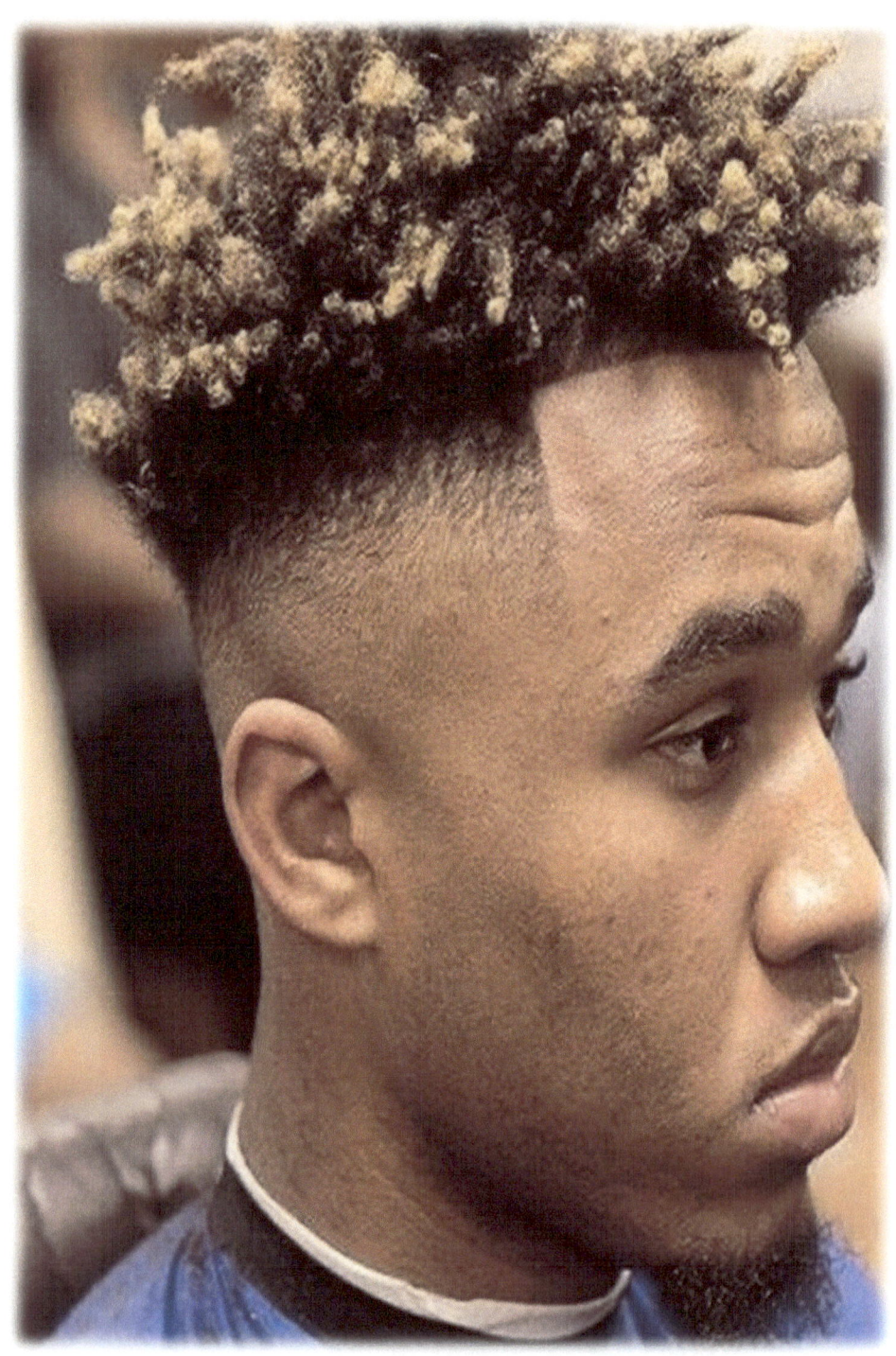

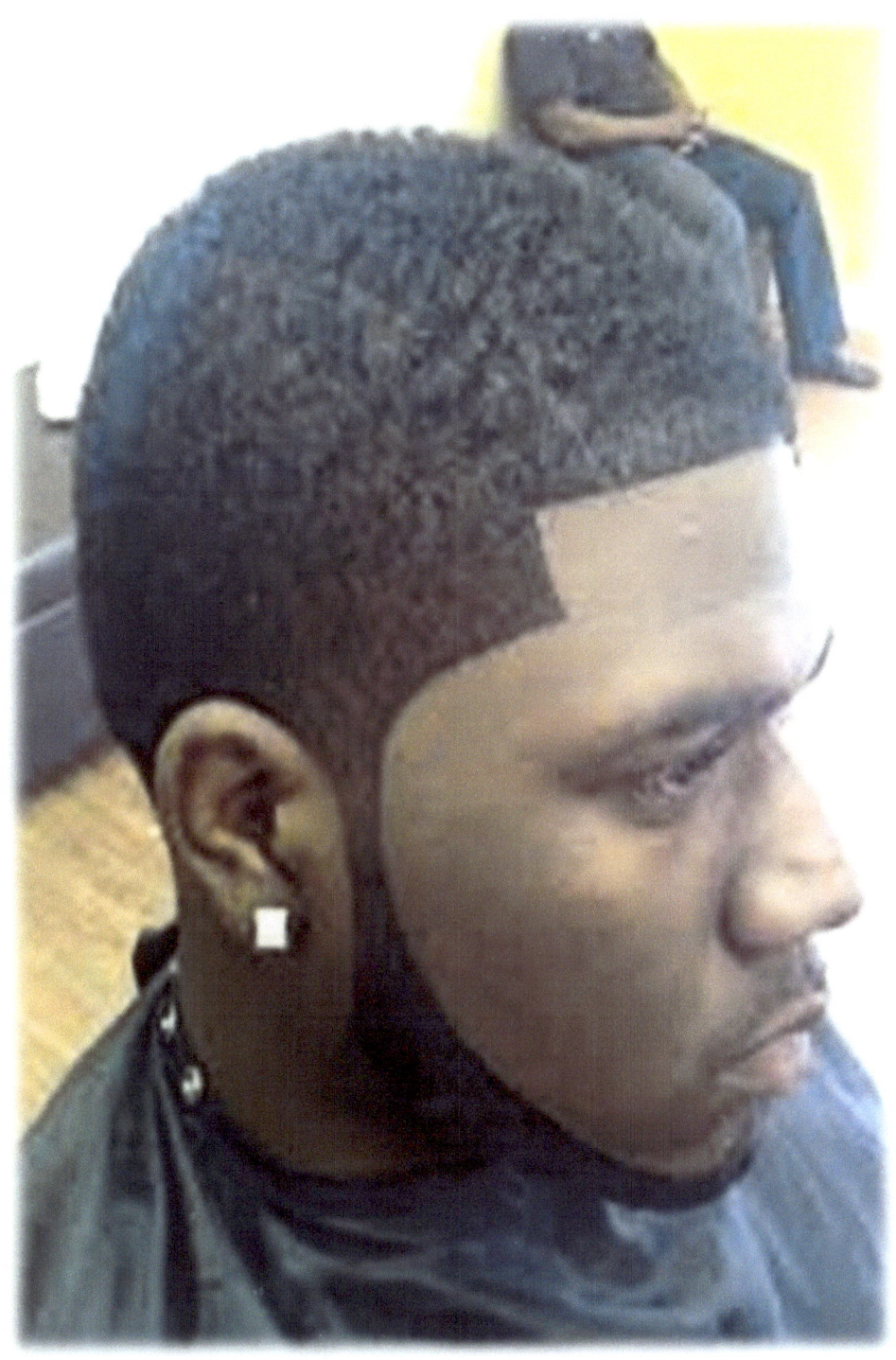

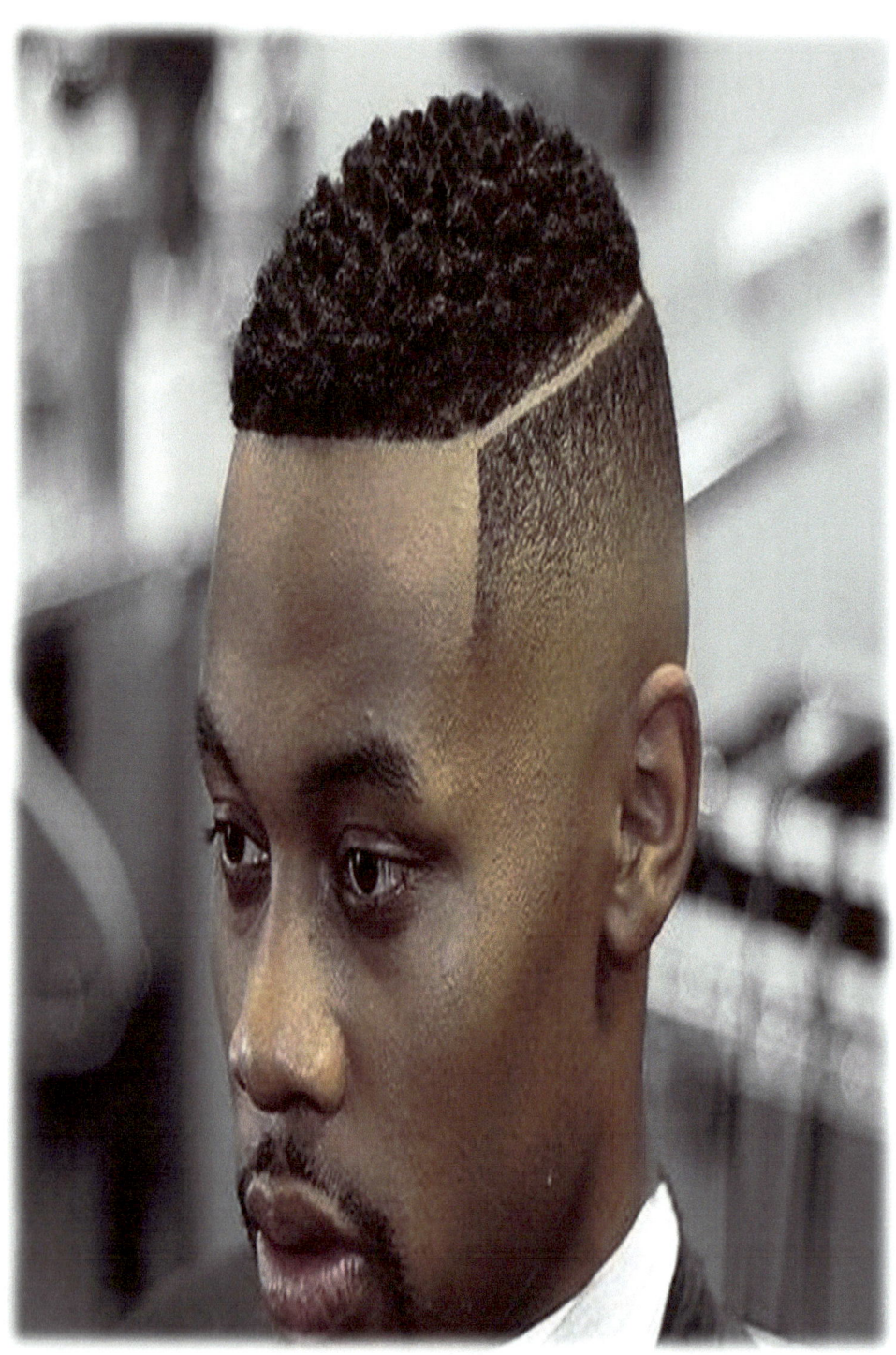

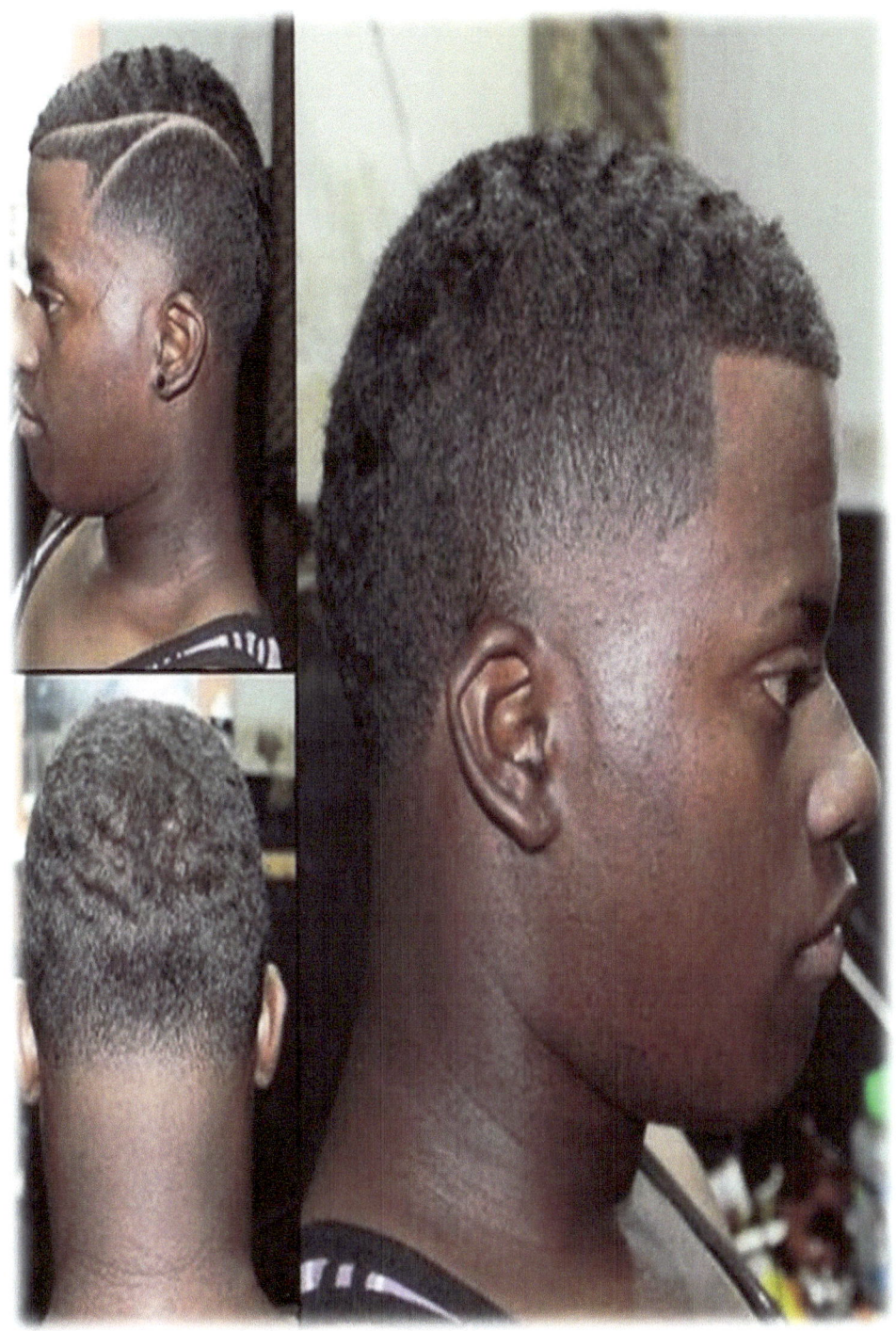

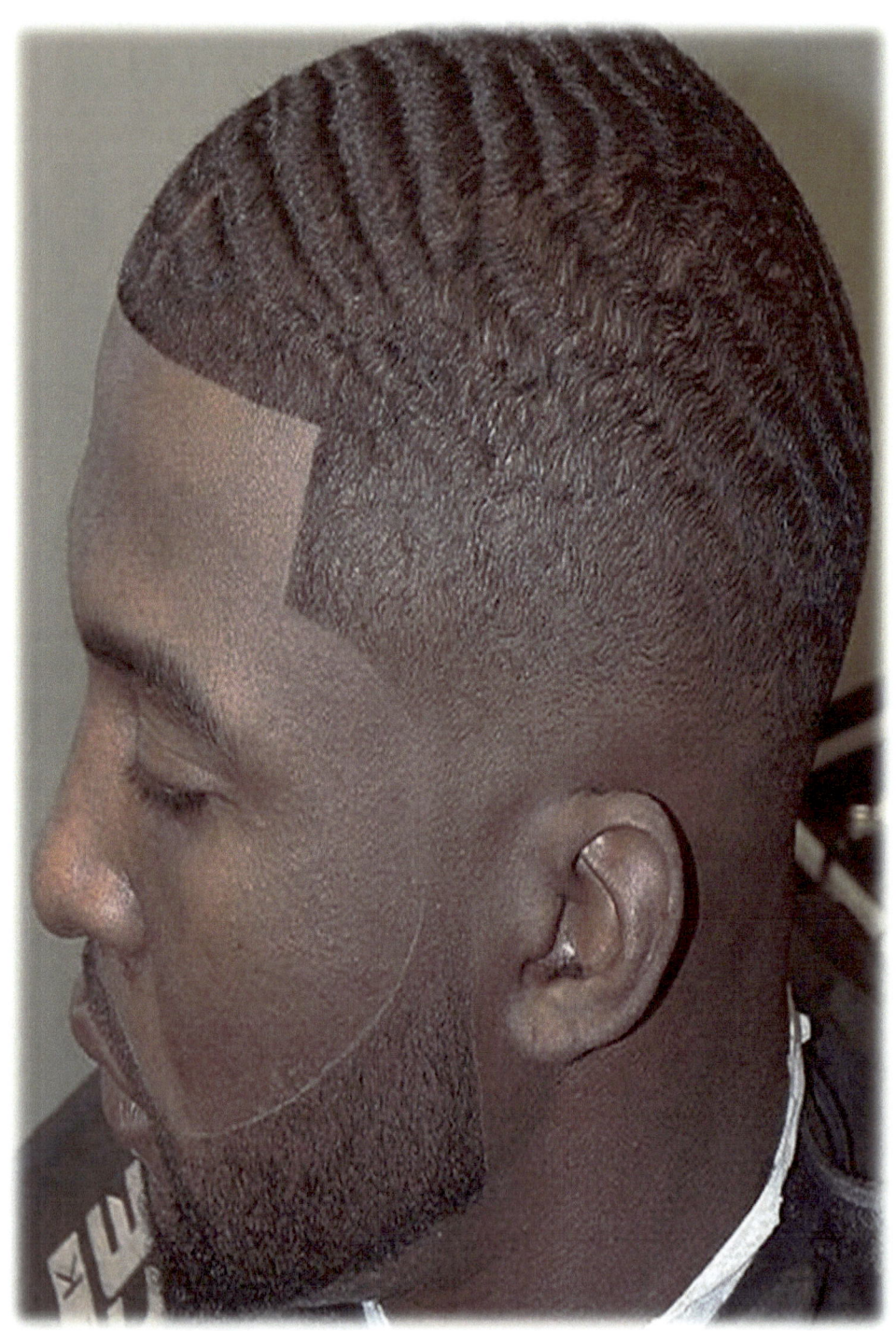

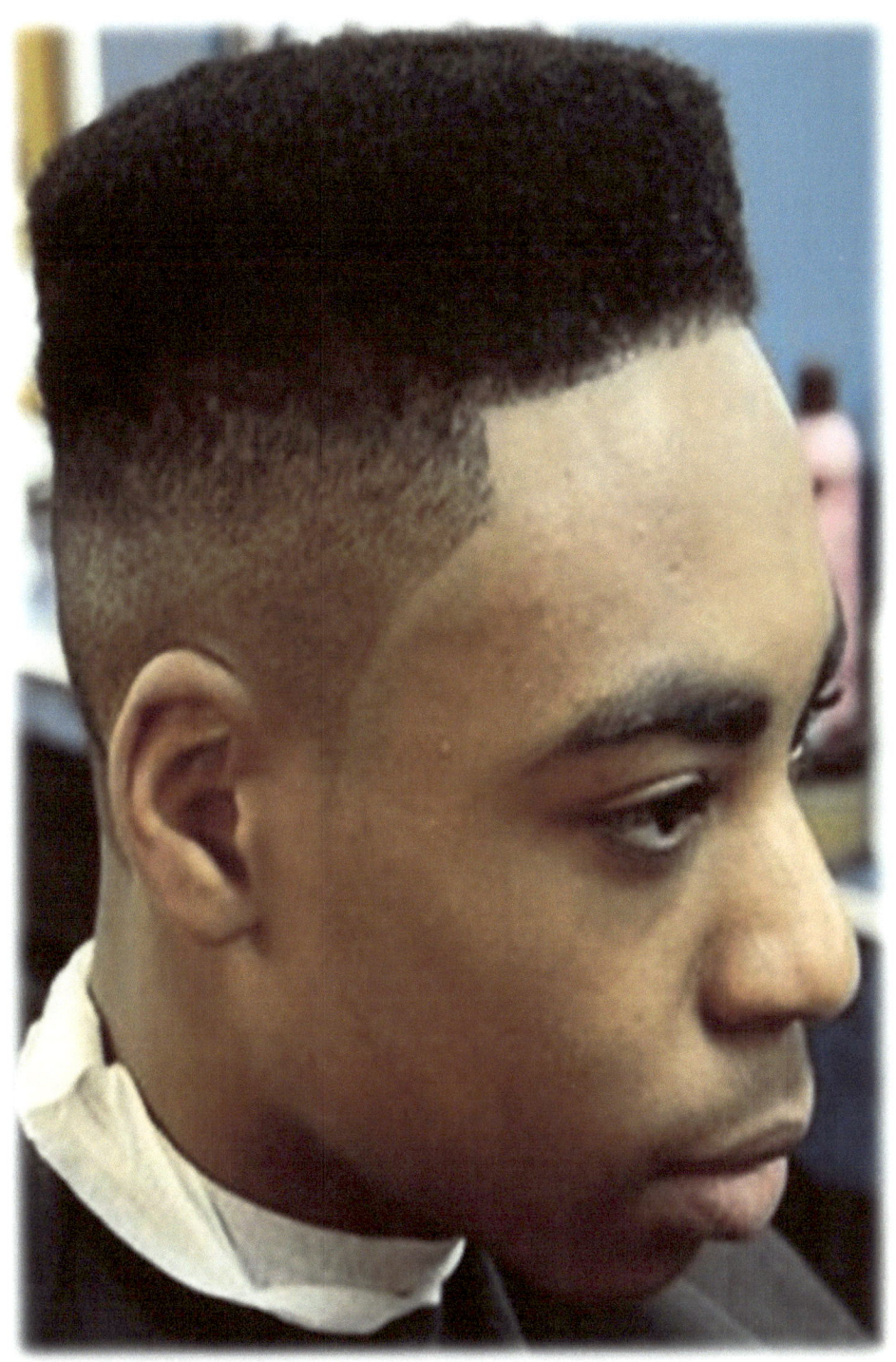

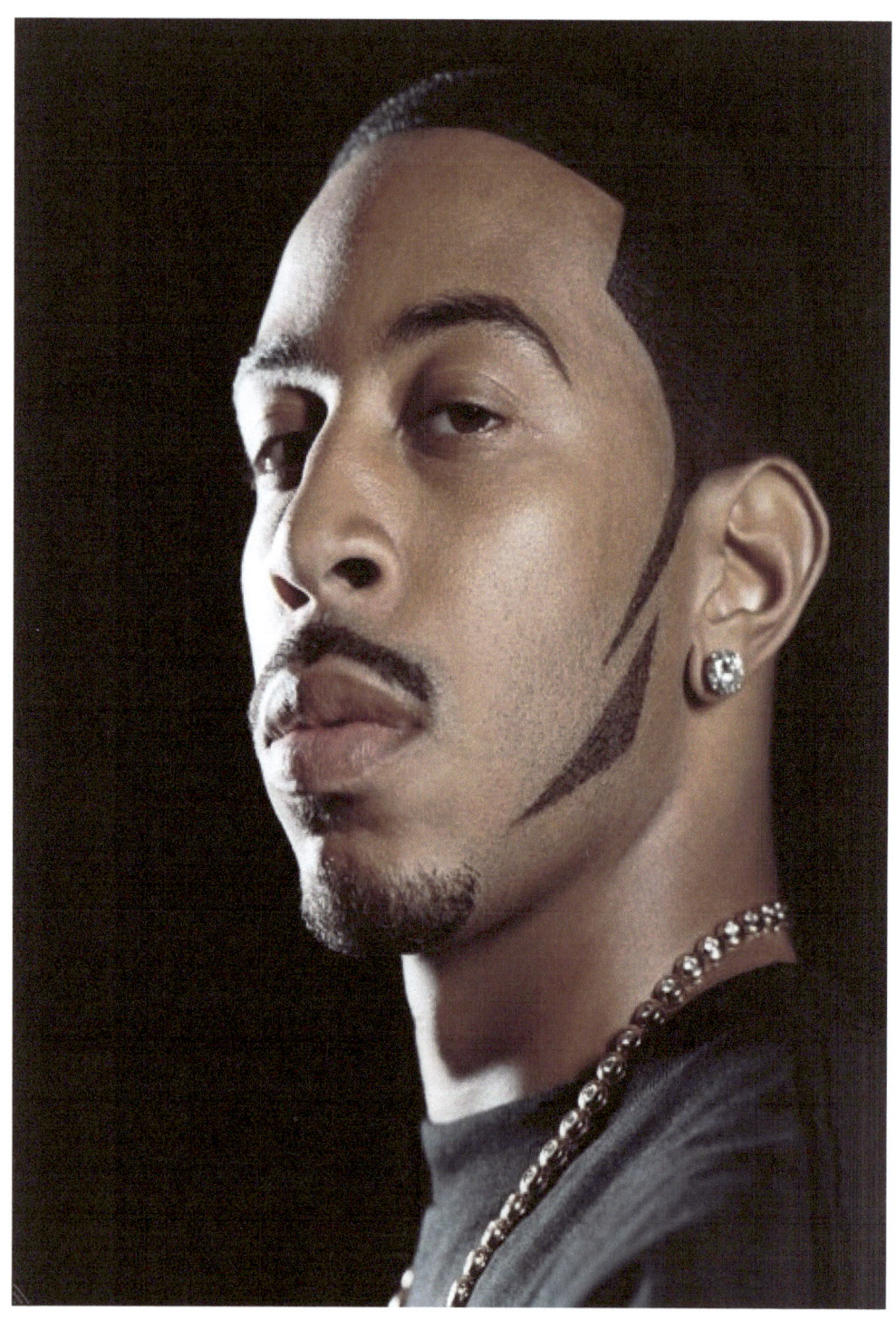

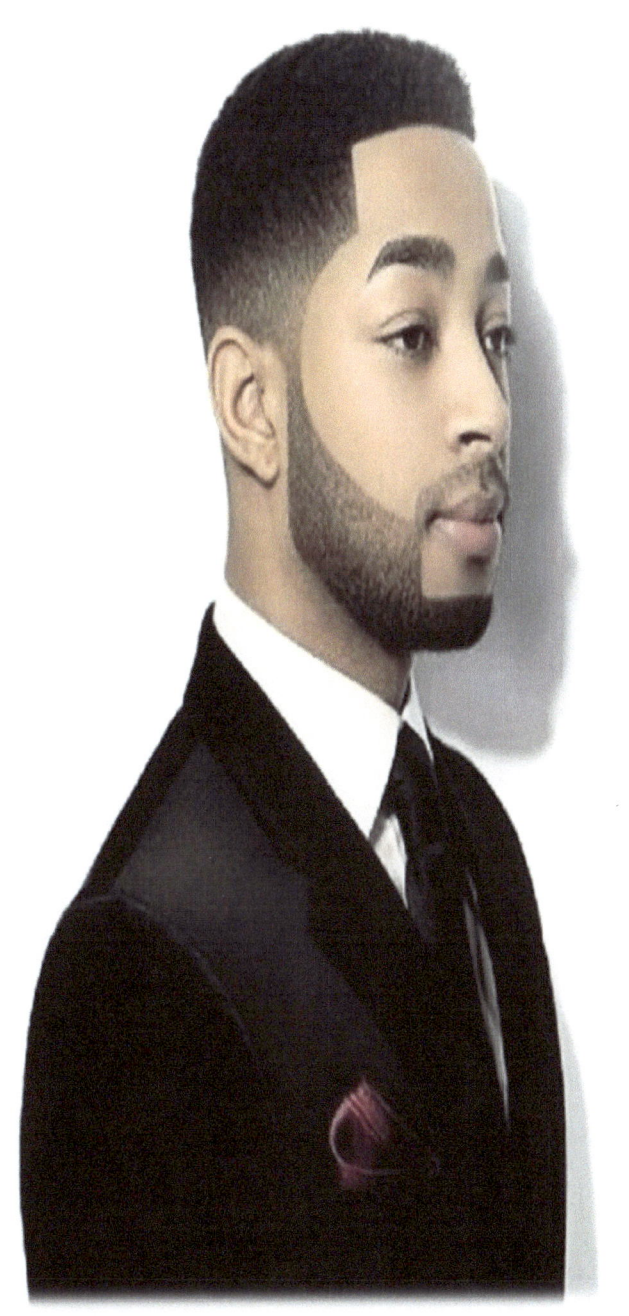

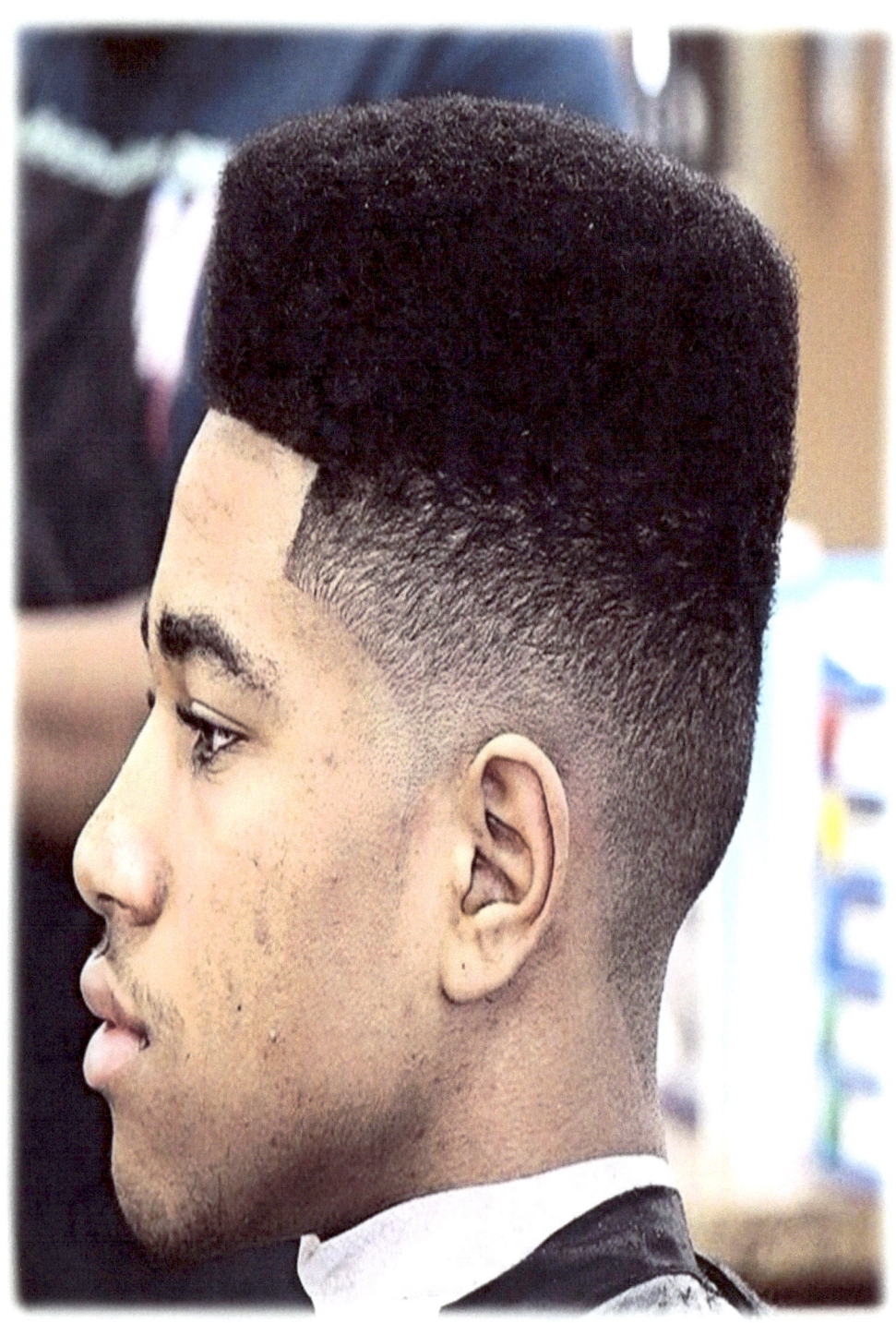

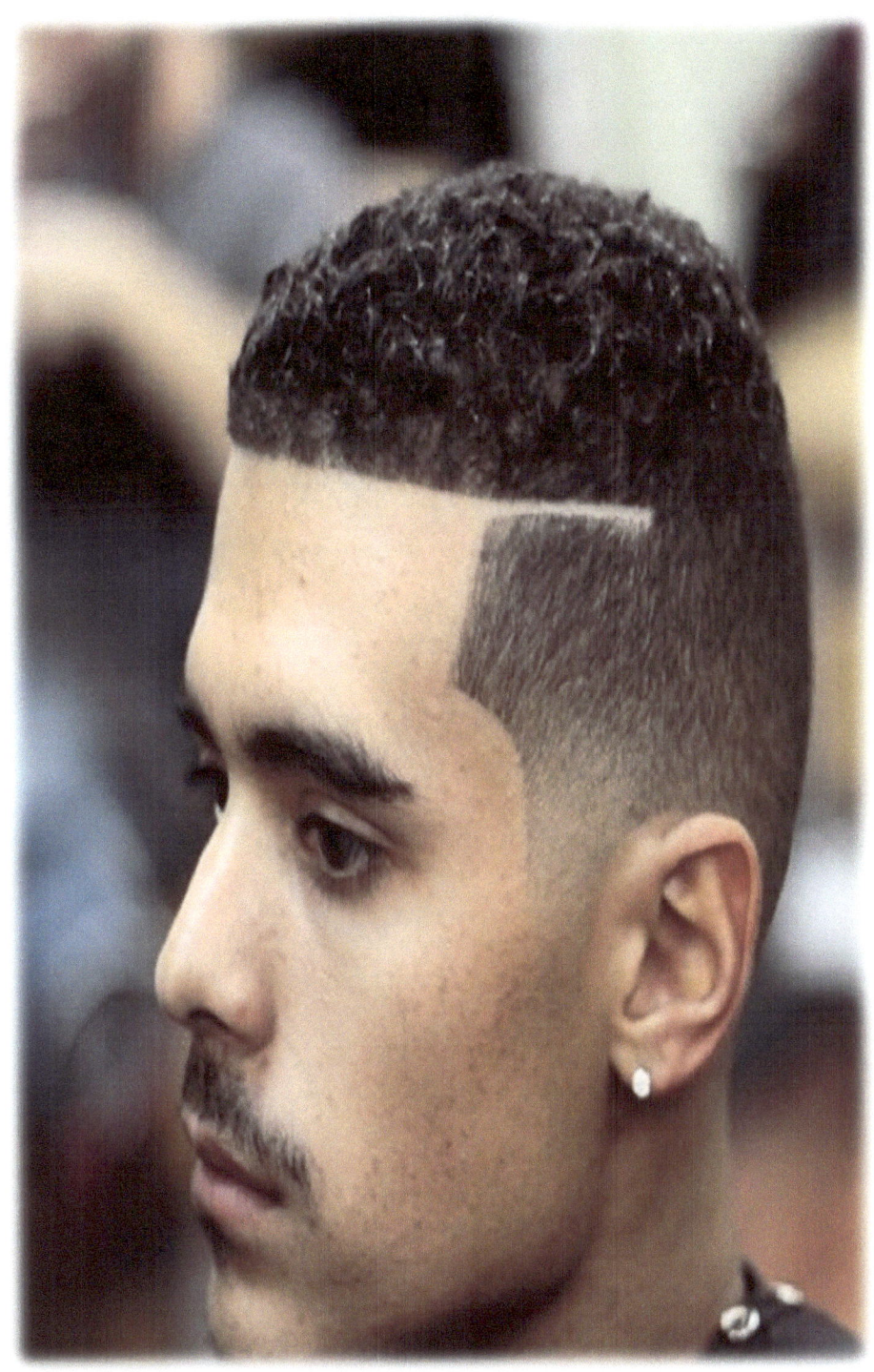

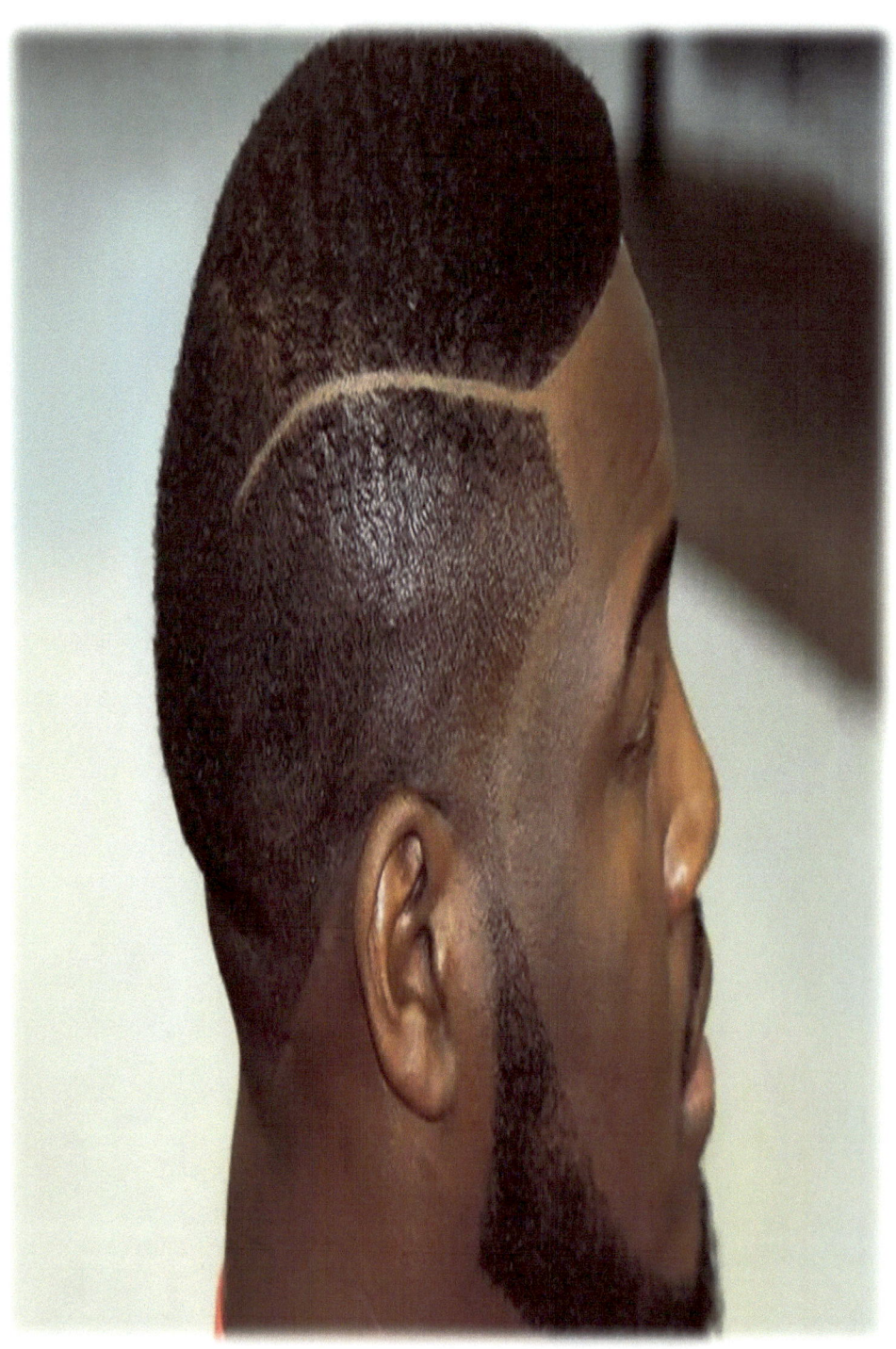

THE ULTIMATE
GENUINE ORIGINAL - PATENT PENDING
MO BROS
EST 2011
LONDON
PREMIUM
SUPERIOR
RAZORS
AFTER SHAVE
LOTION

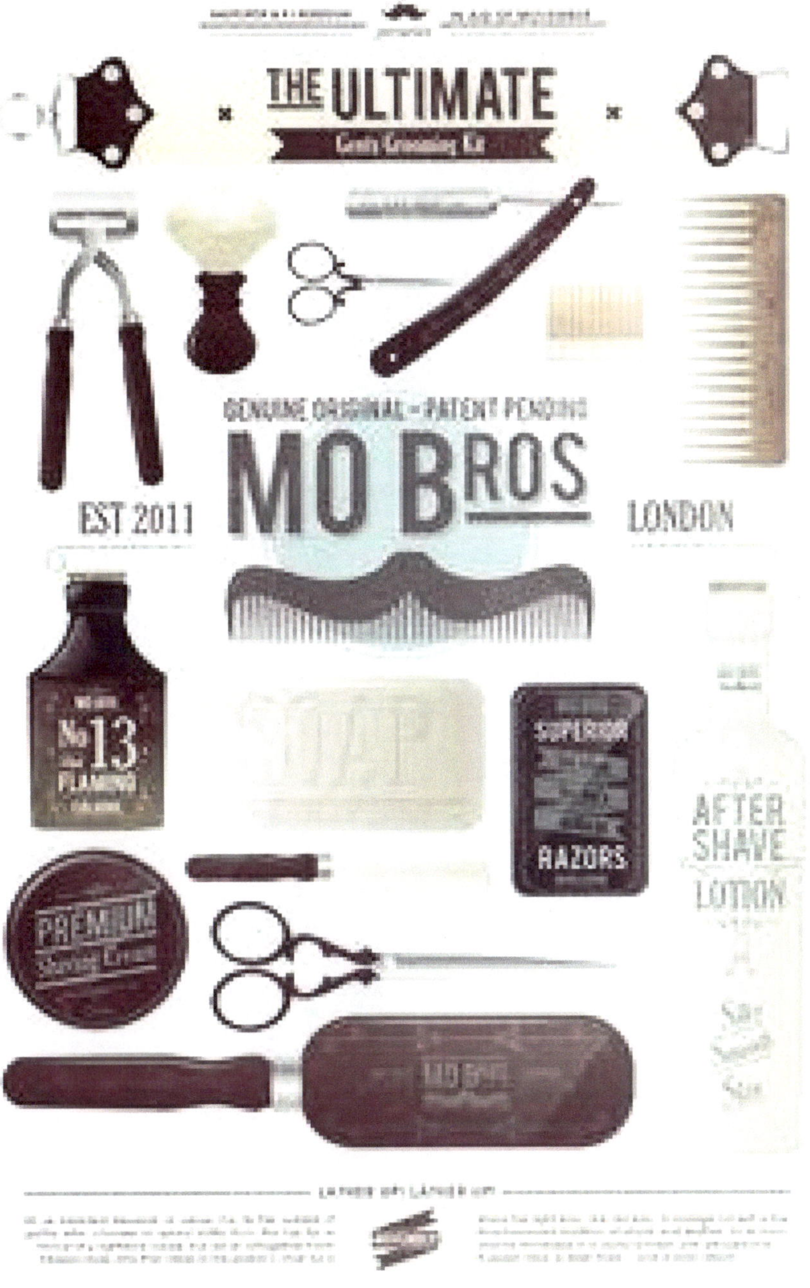

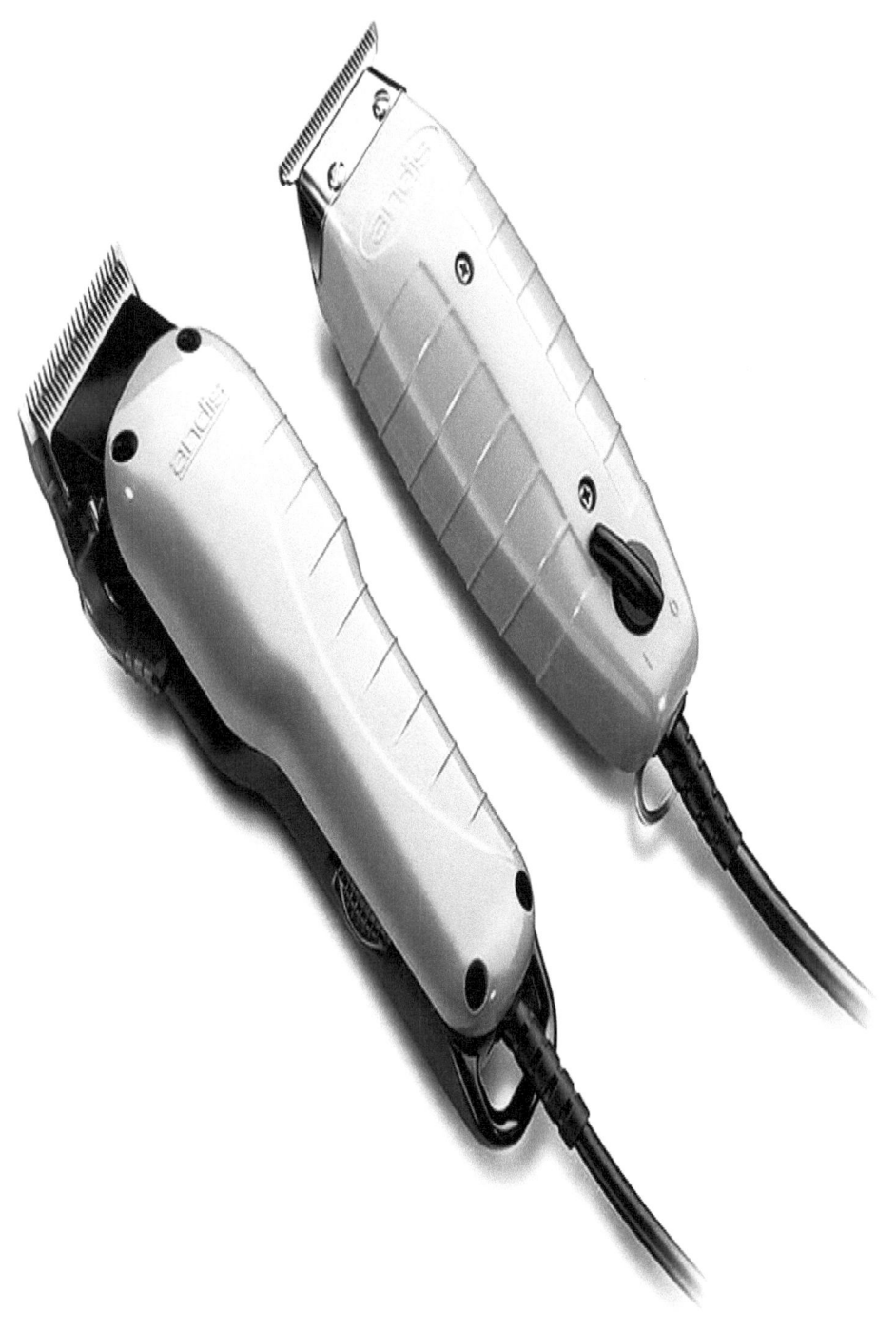

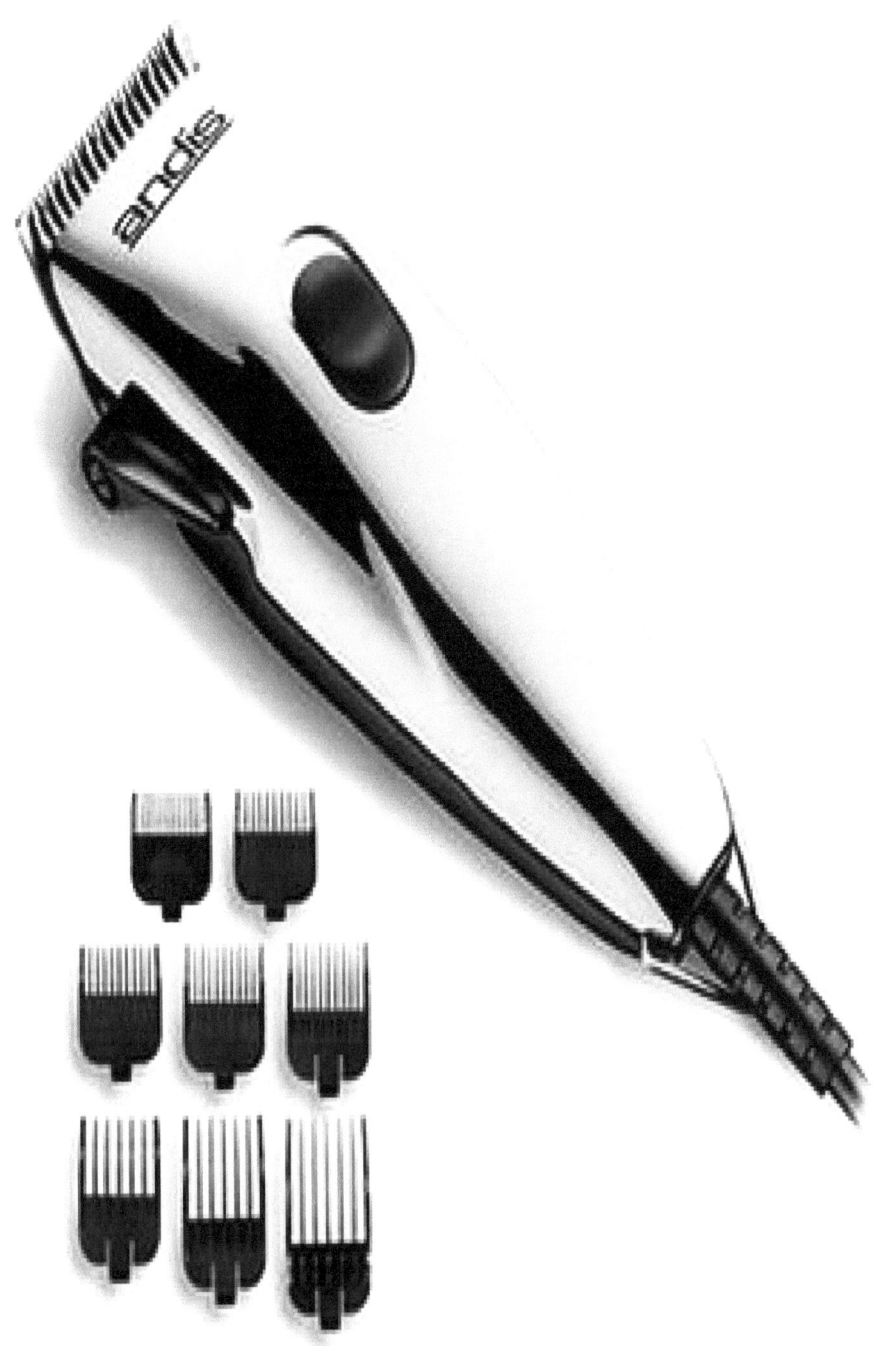

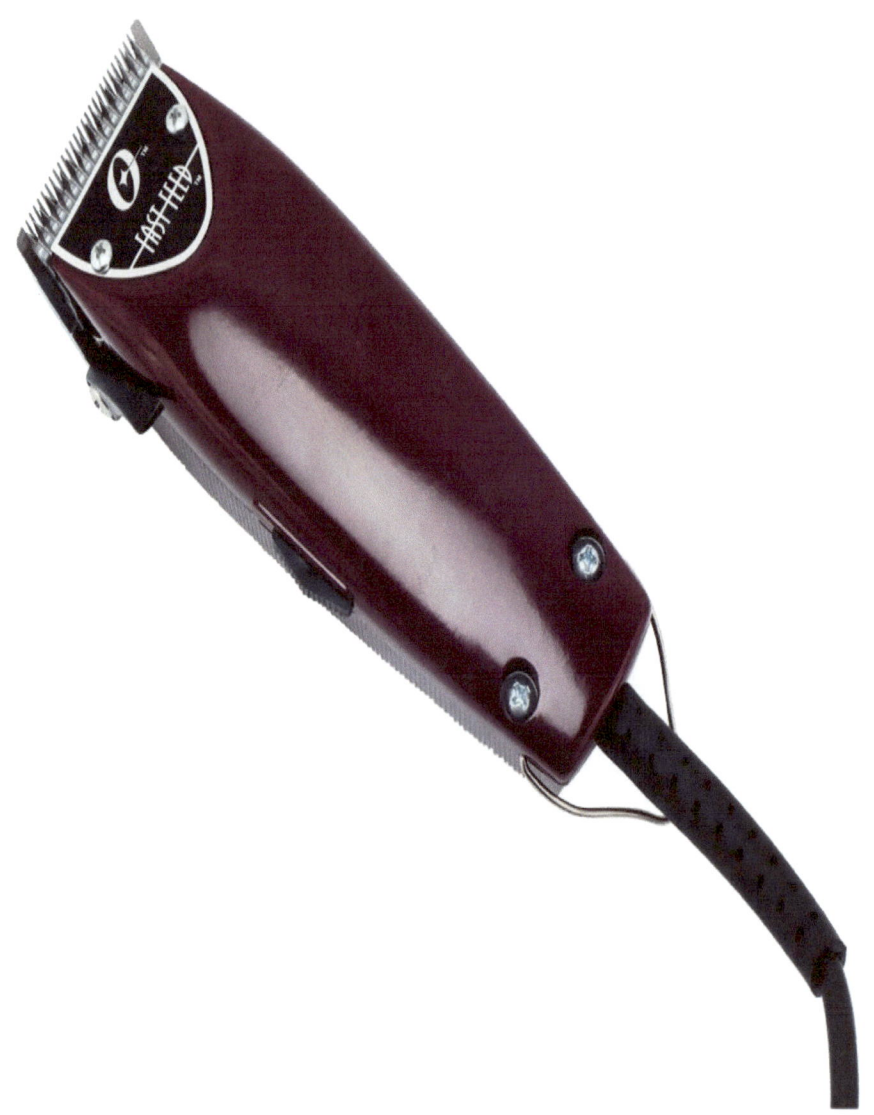

Forget yesterday.

It has already forgotten you.

Don't sweat tomorrow.

You haven't even met.

Instead, open your eyes,

and your heart to a

truly precious gift;

today.

5 *Quick Ways to Build your Clientele*

1. Hand flyers and business cards in person to future clients
2. Word of mouth
3. Social media
4. Offer regular clients a discount for bringing you new clients
5. Special Offer on services

Tips for the Barbershop and Beauty Salon

1. Cleanliness is important in the establishment

2. Communication is important with clients

3. Do not talk about your personal life with clients

4. Do not bring drama to the establishment

5. Do not keep clients waiting

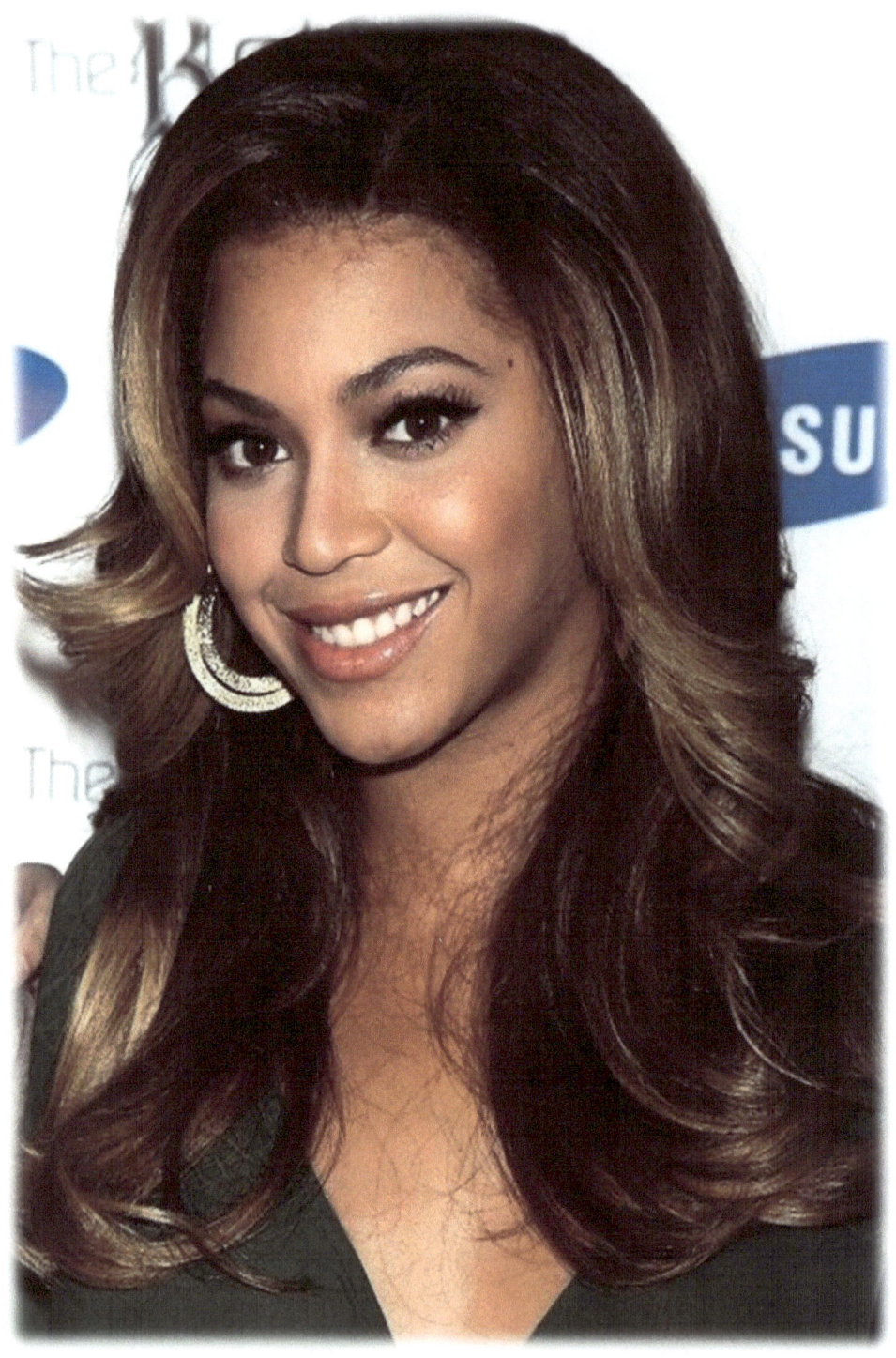

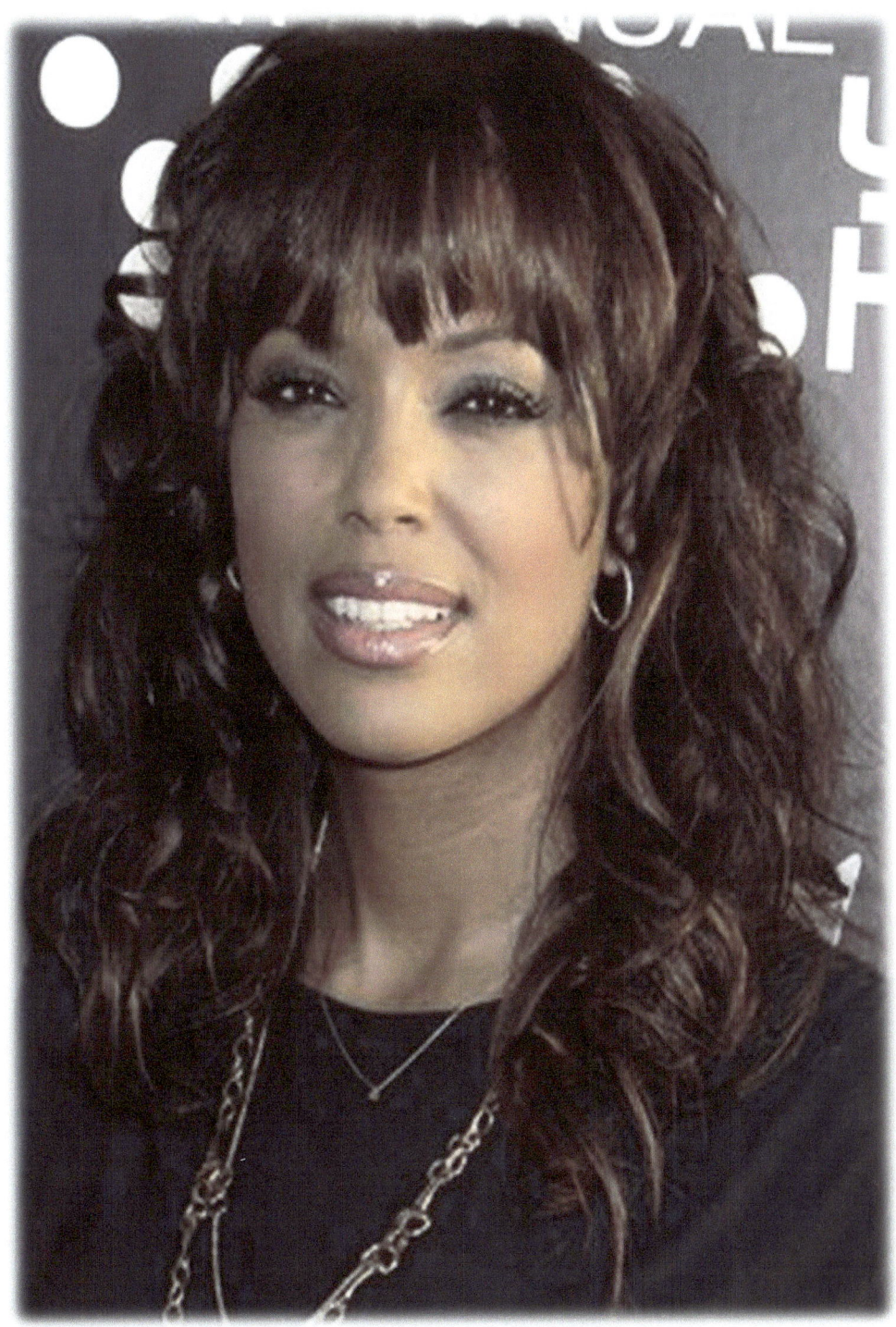

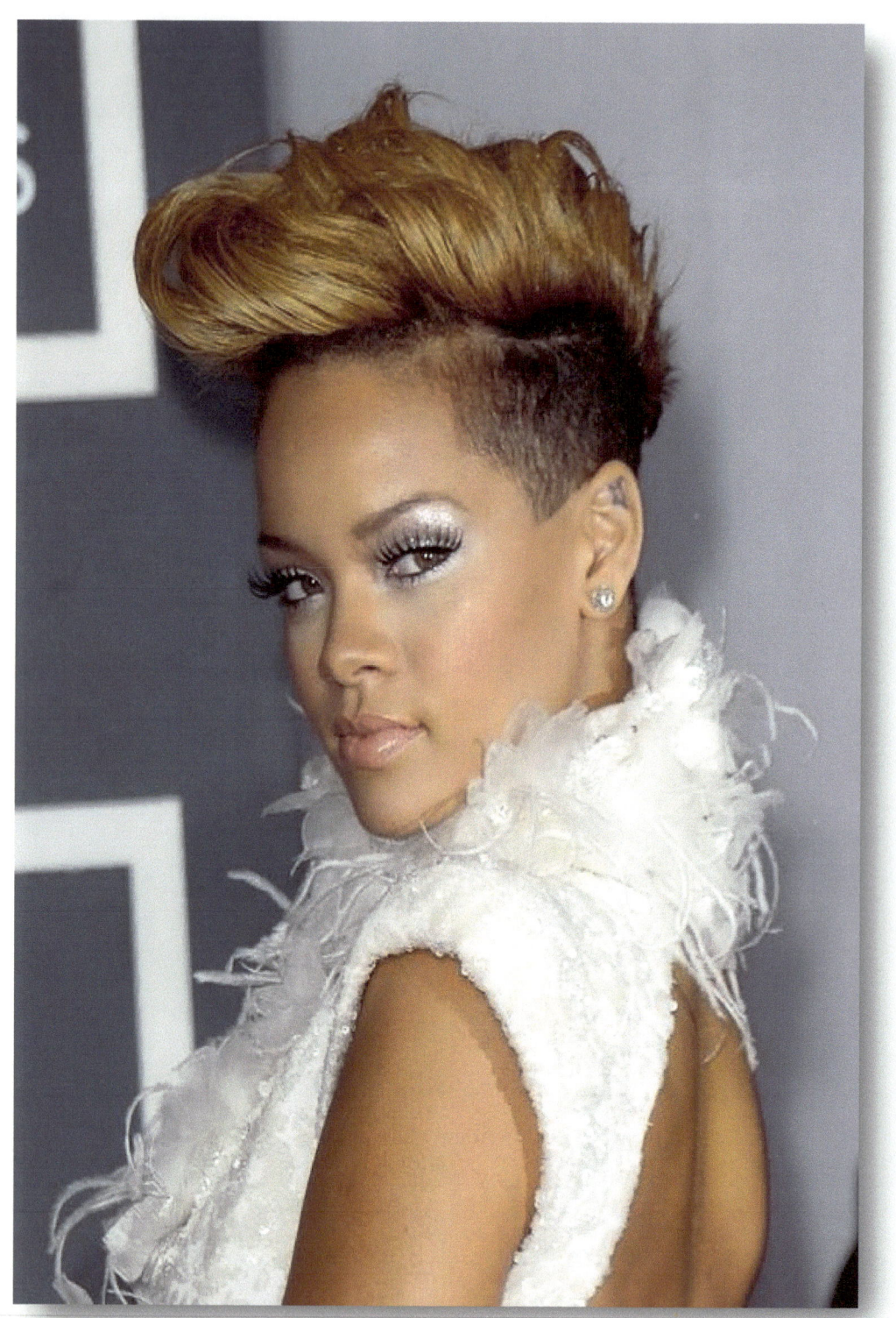

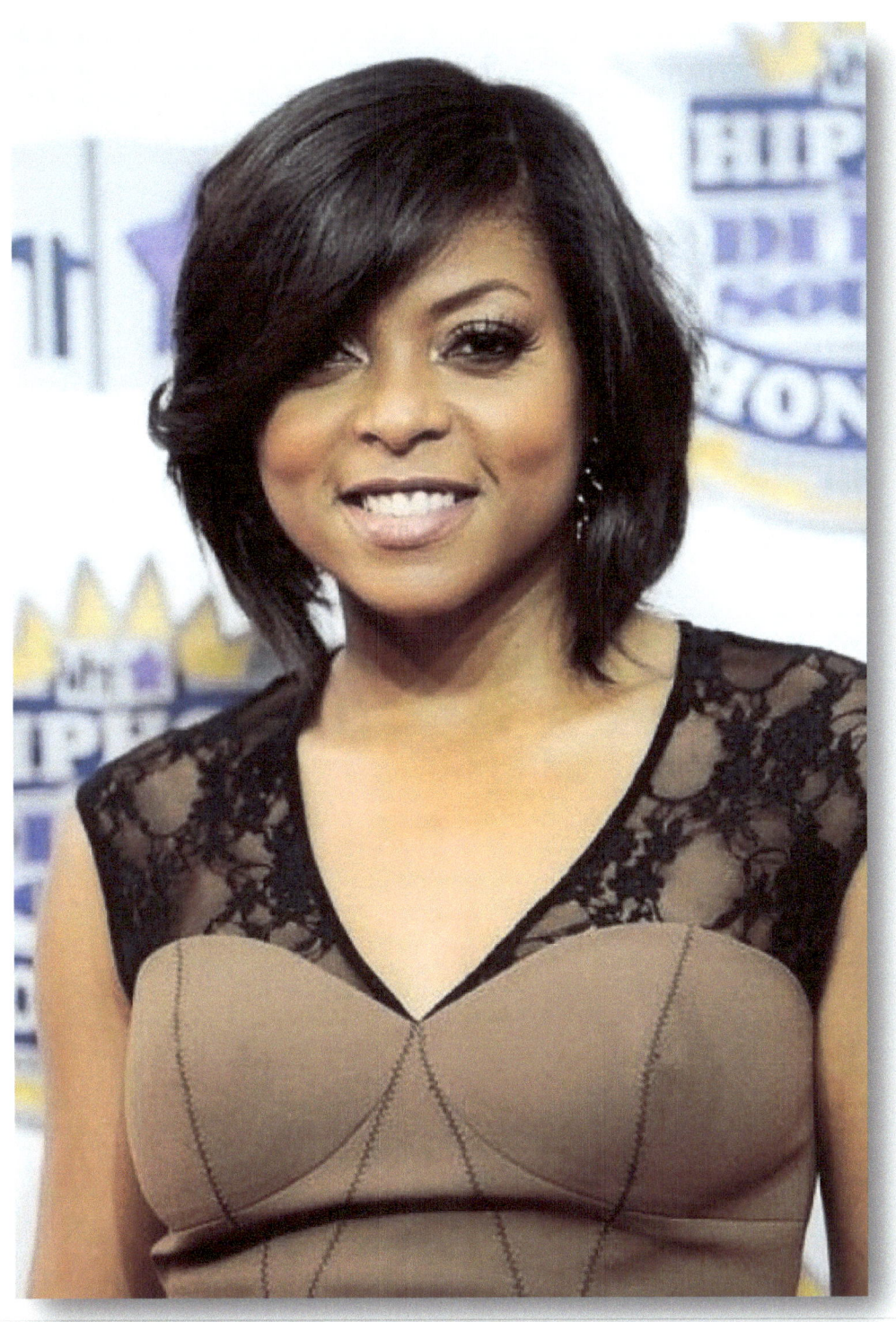

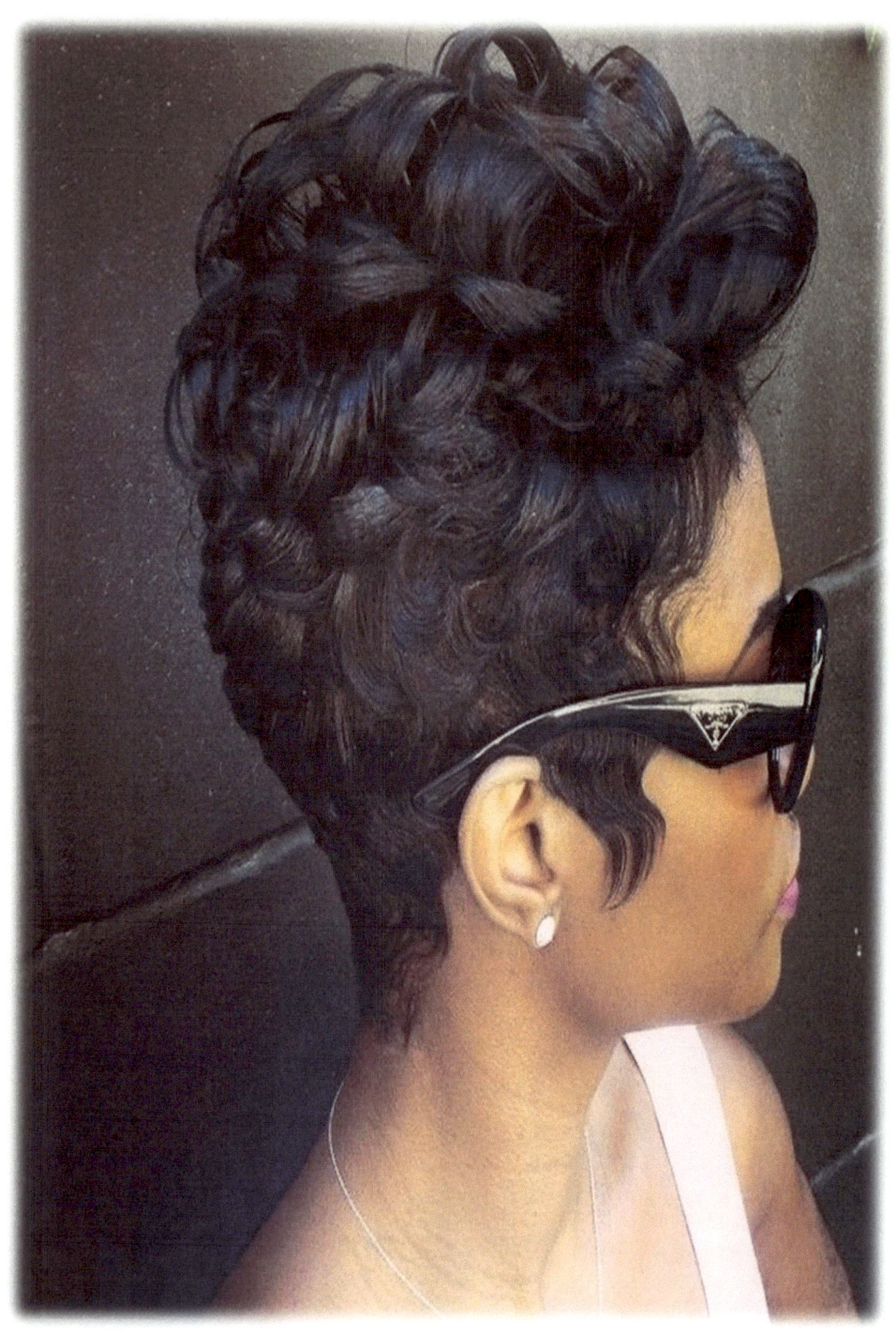

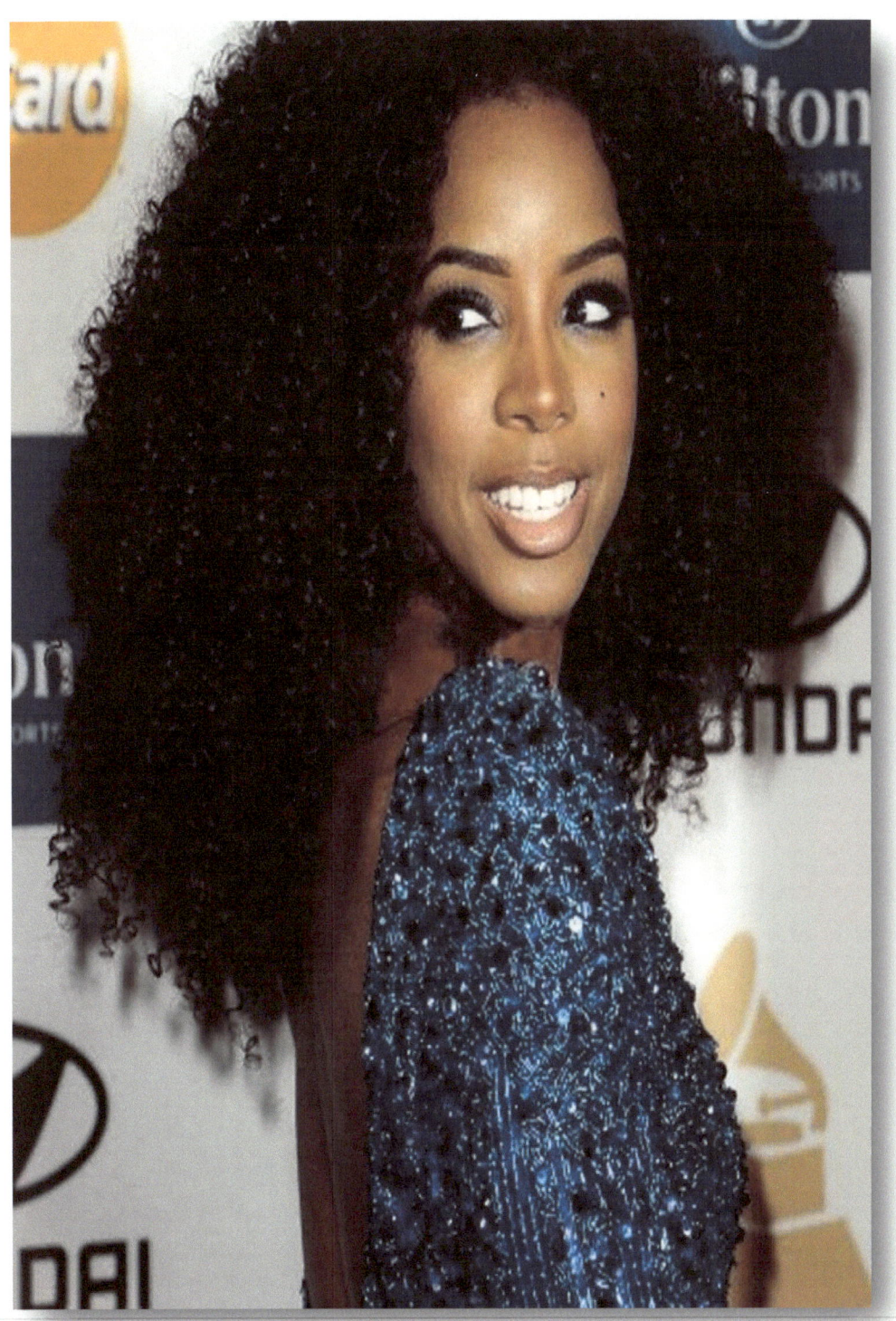

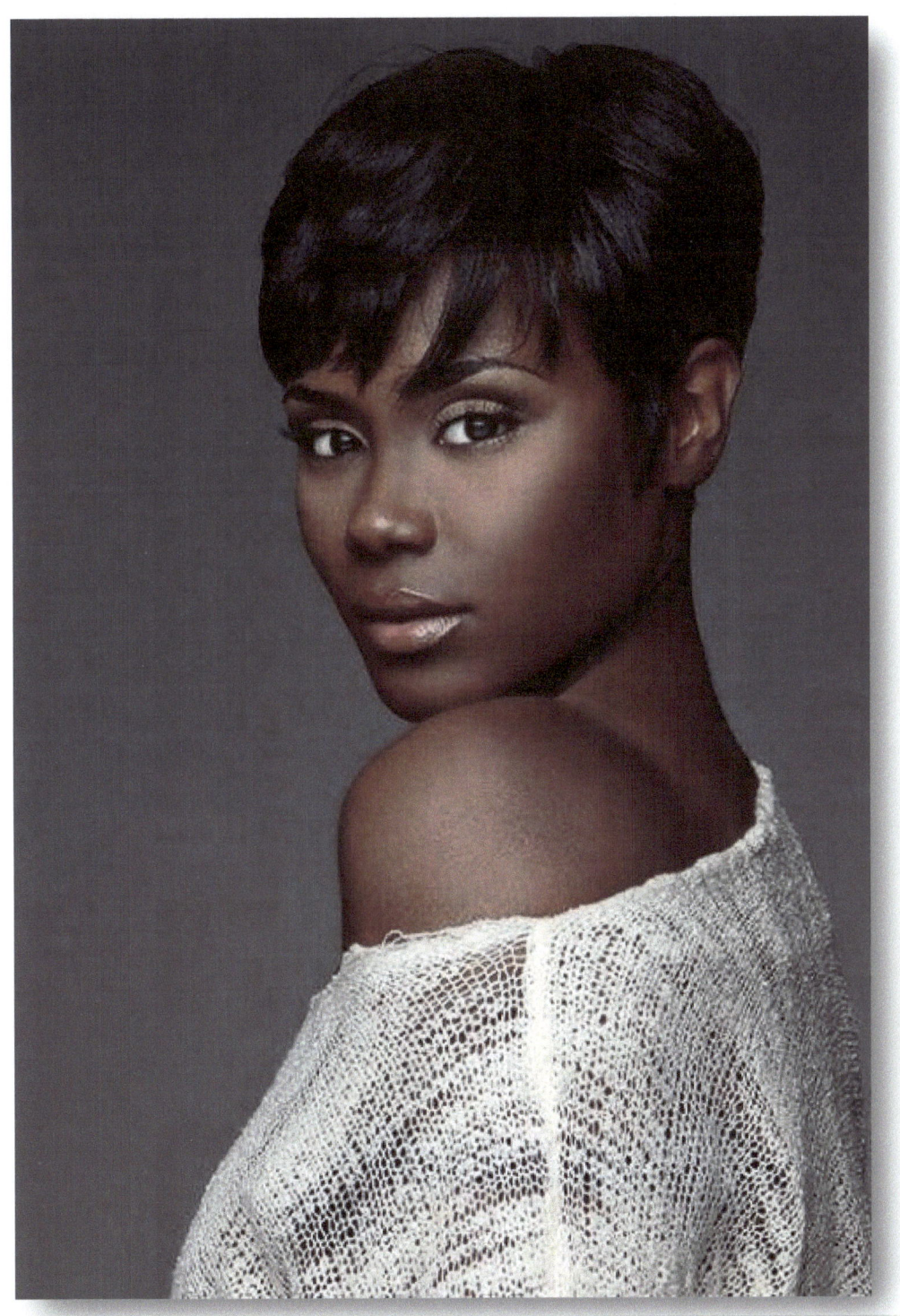

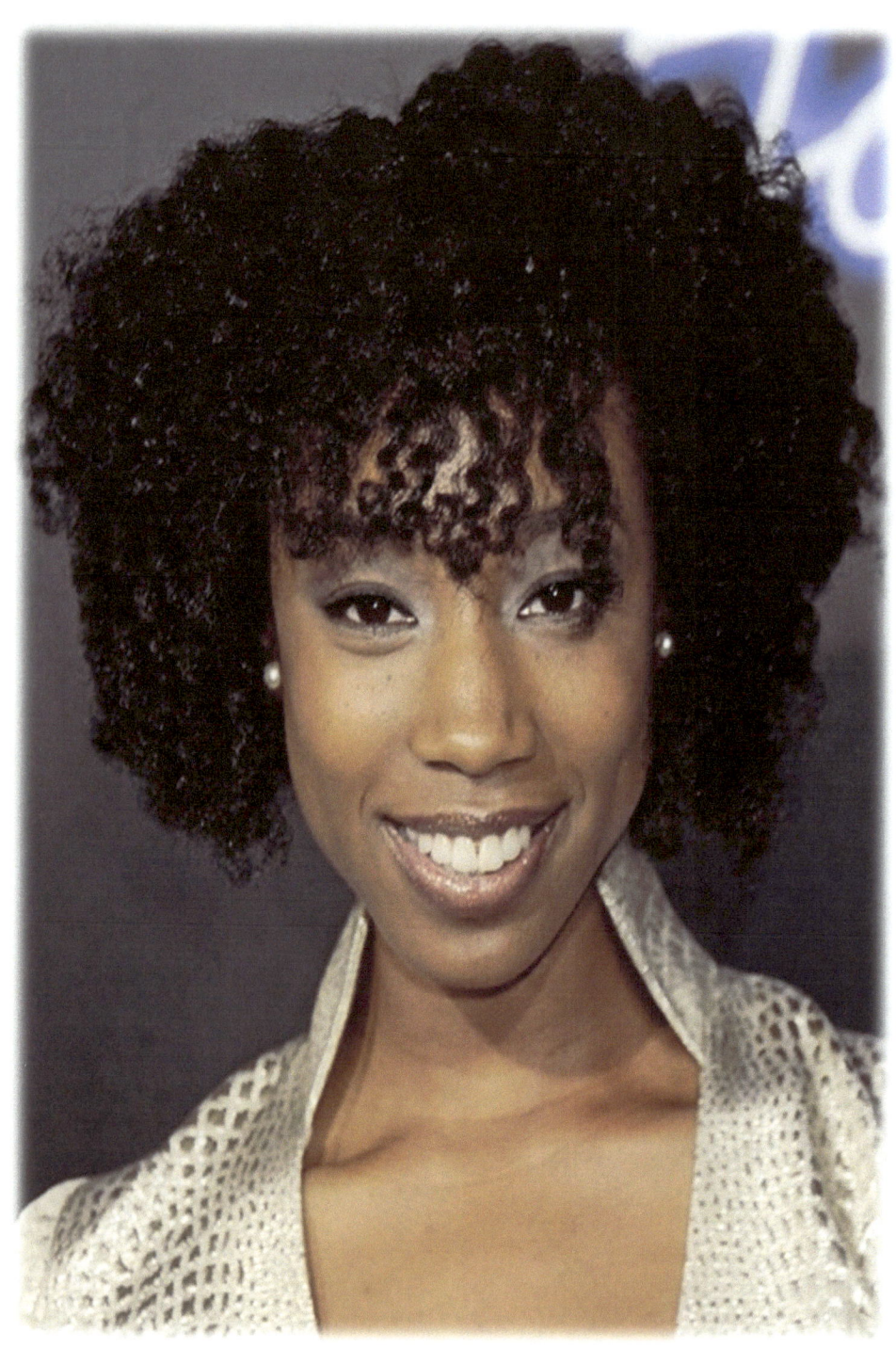

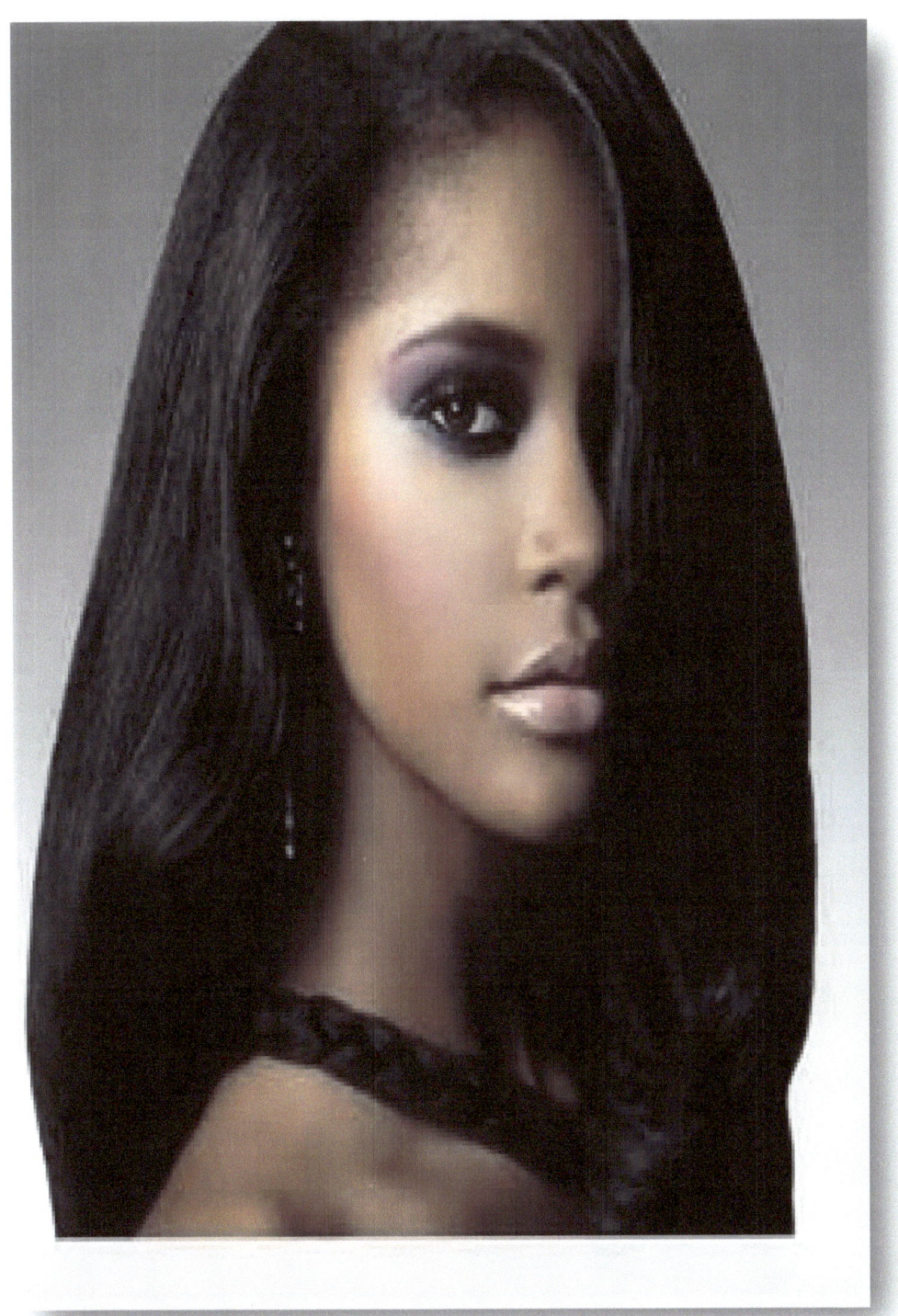

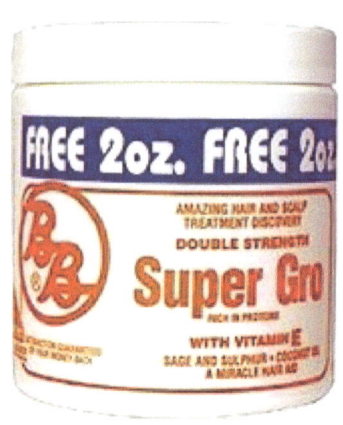

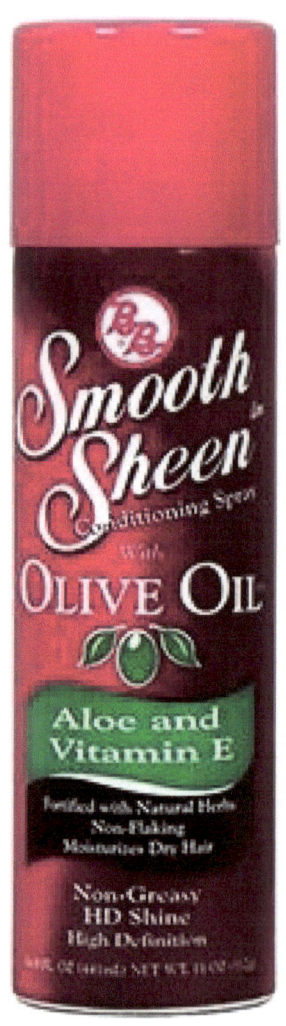

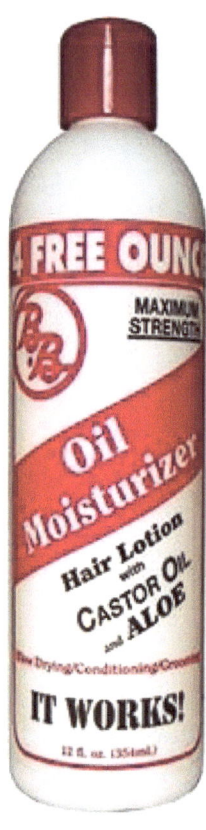

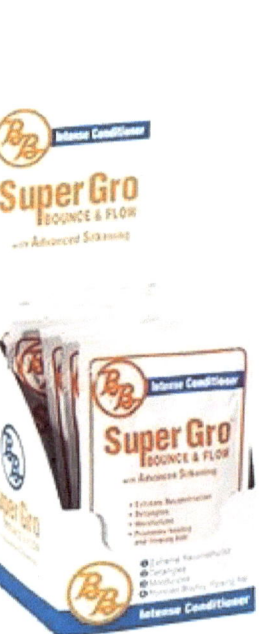

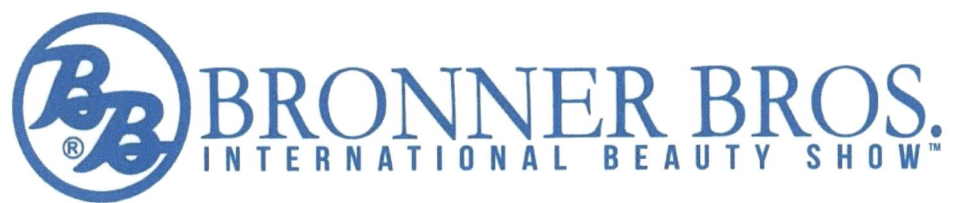

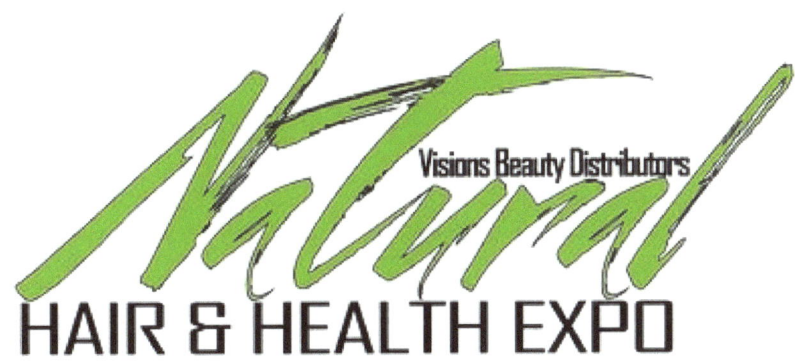

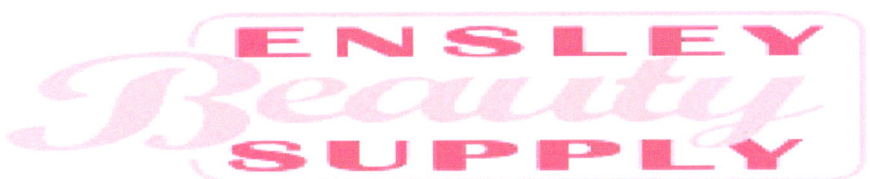

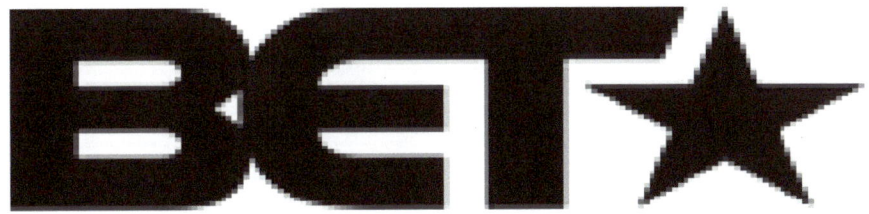

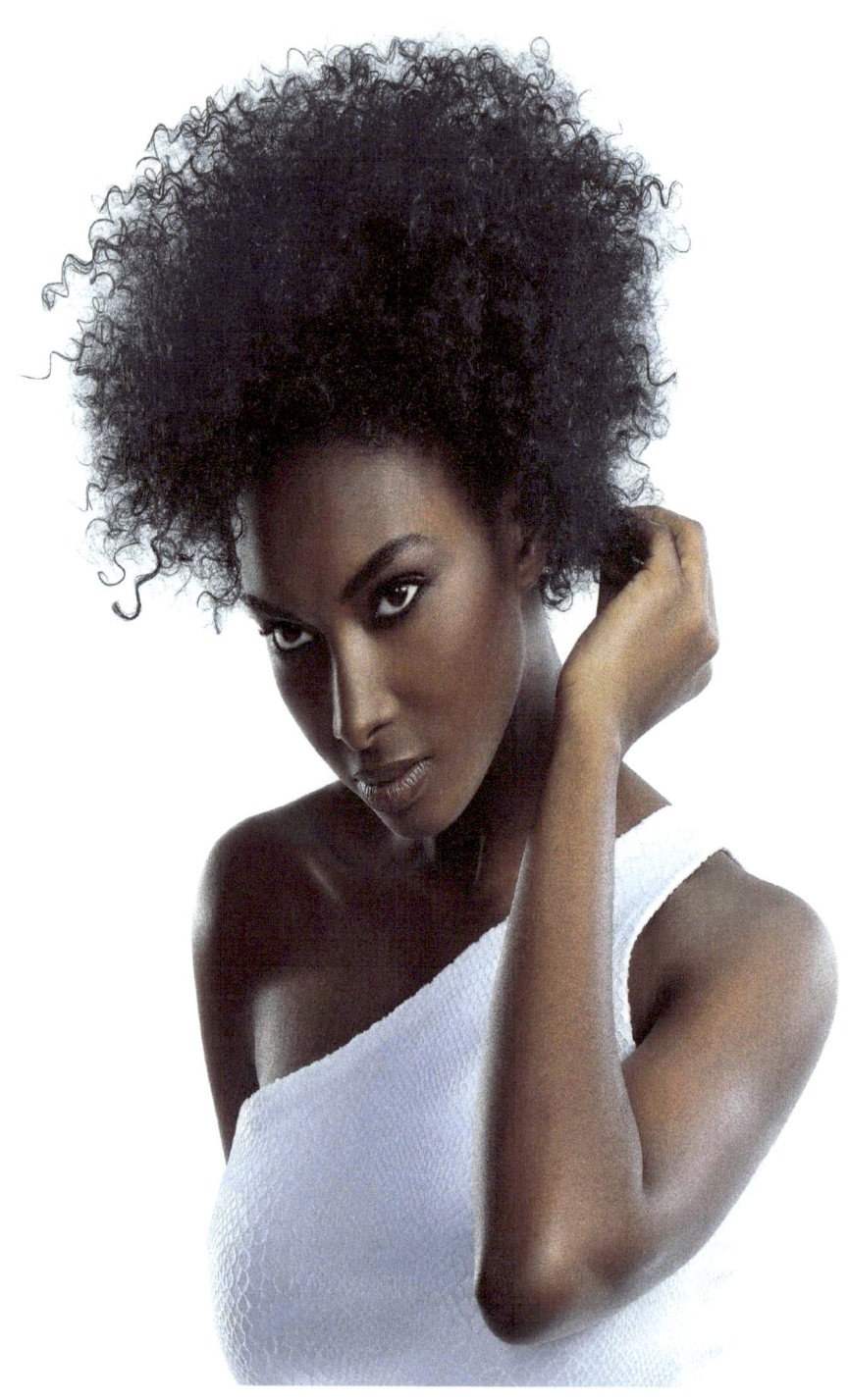

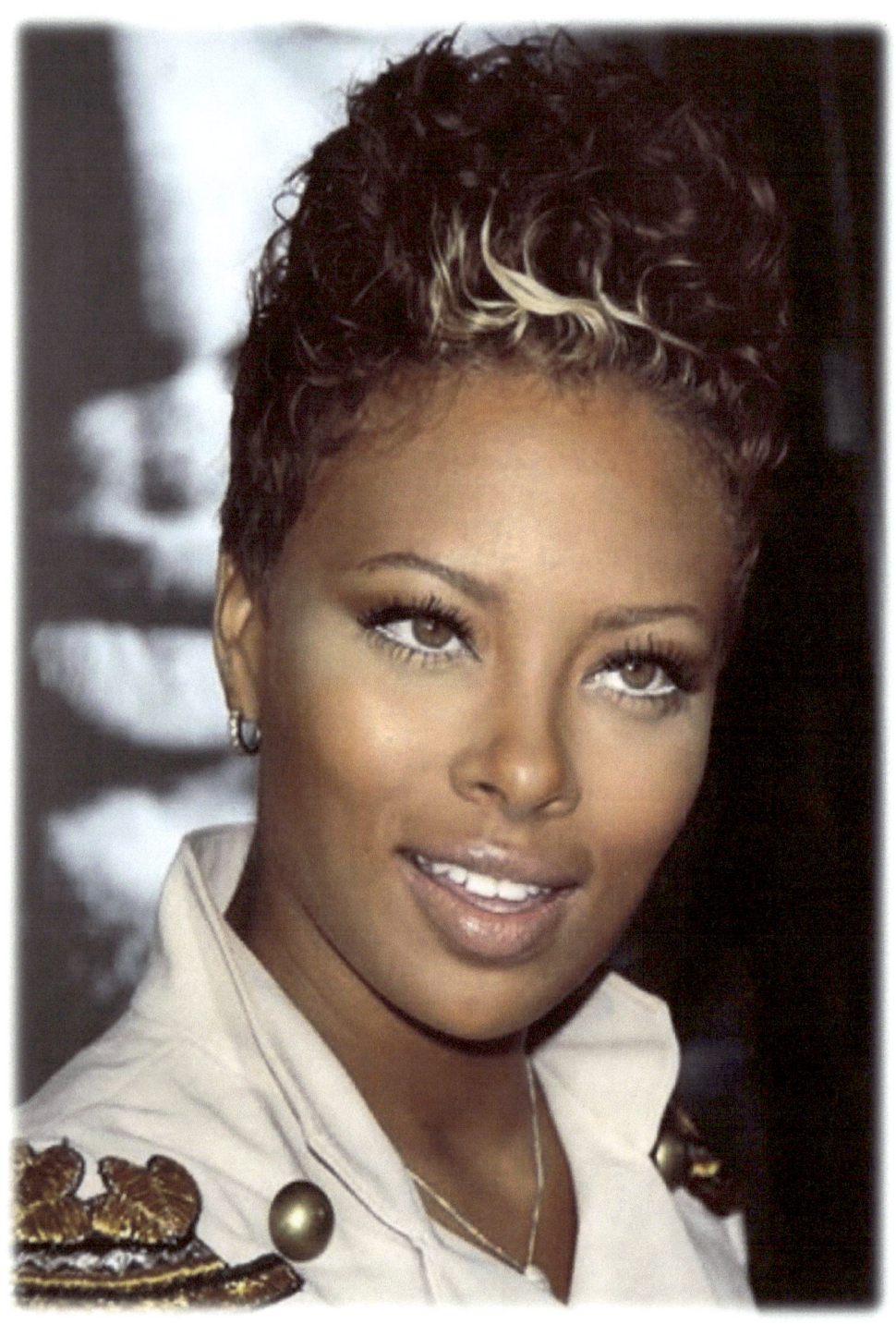

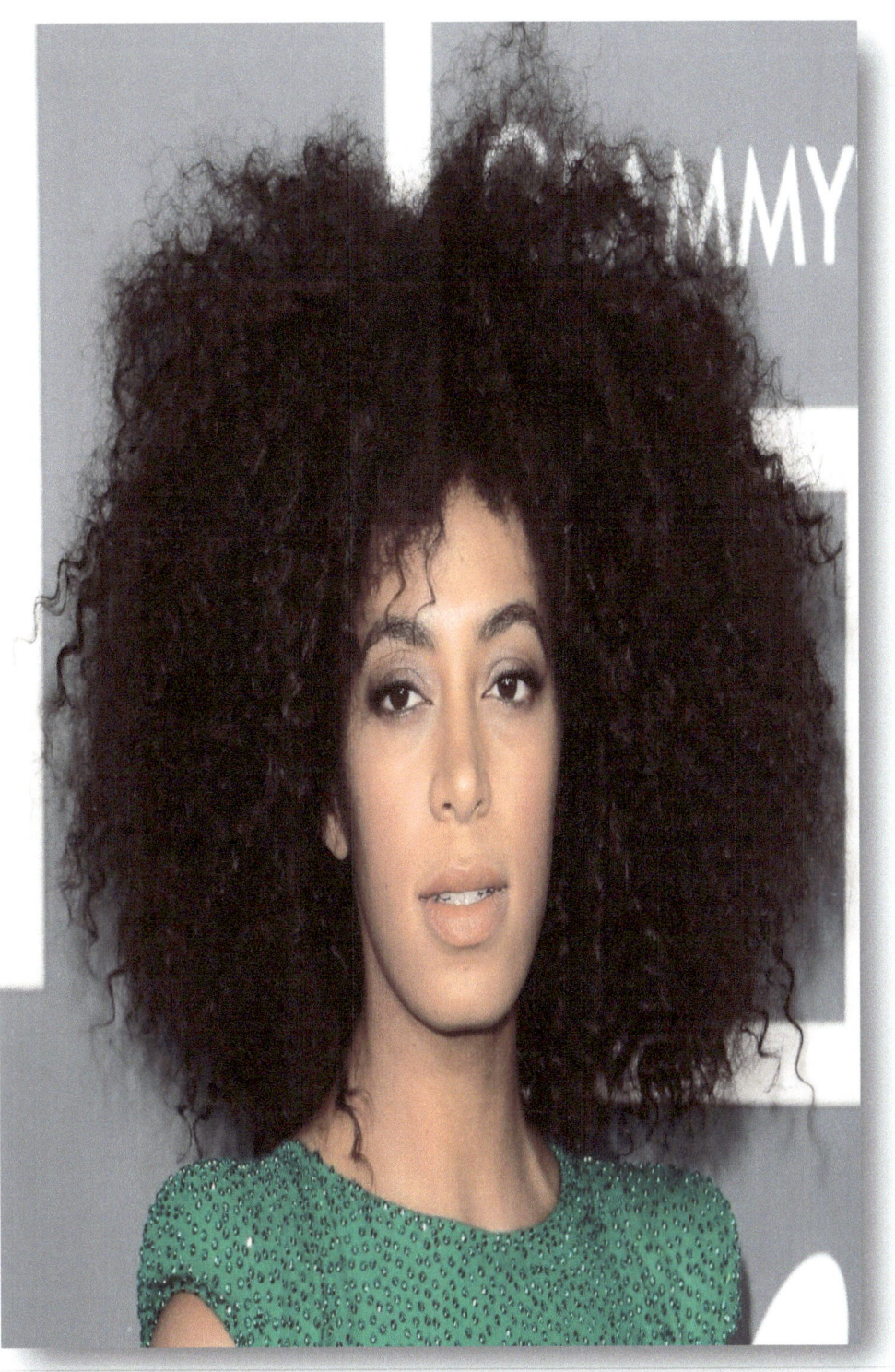

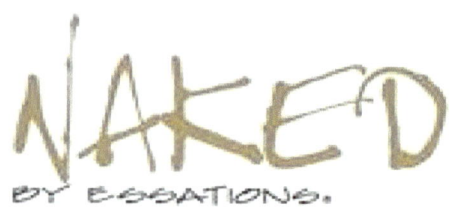

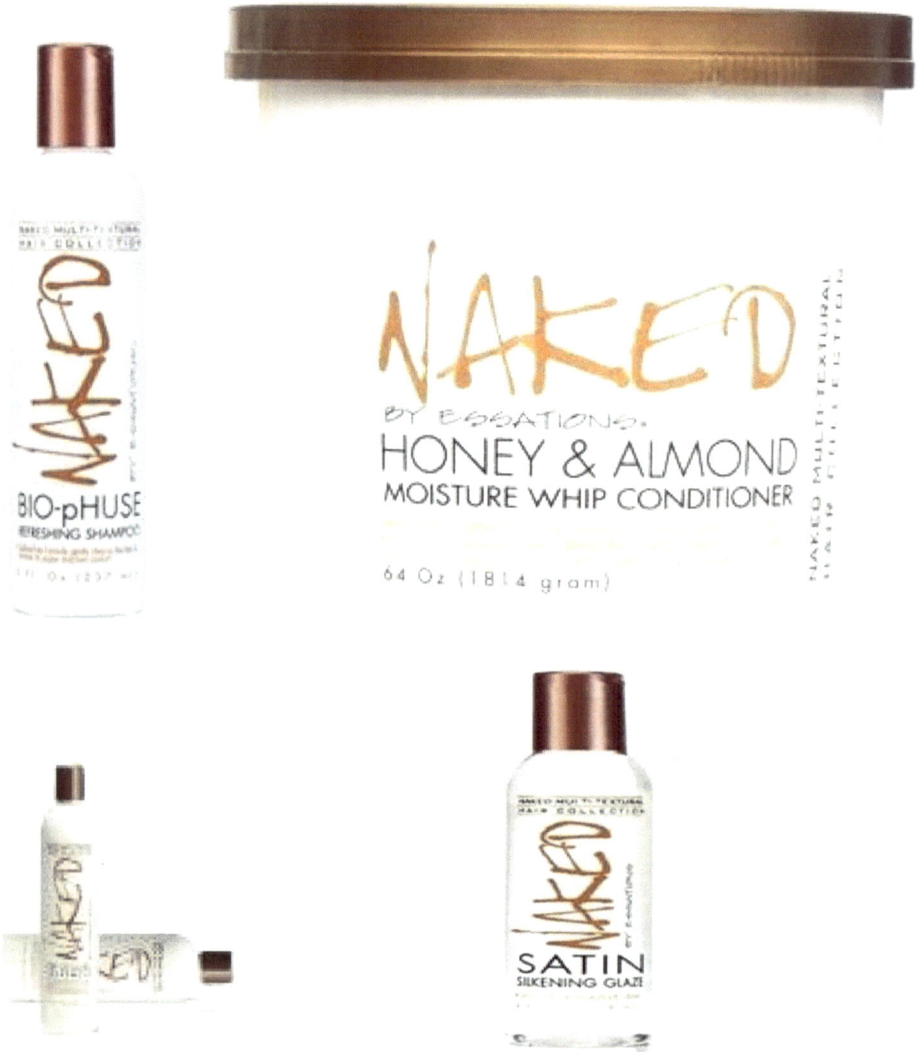

NAKED

BY ESSATIONS.

NAKED
BIO-pHUSE
REFRESHING SHAMPOO
NAKED
BY ESSATIONS.
HONEY & ALMOND
MOISTURE WHIP CONDITIONER
64 Oz (1814 gram)
NAKED MULTI-TEXTURAL
NAKED
SATIN
SILKENING GLAZE

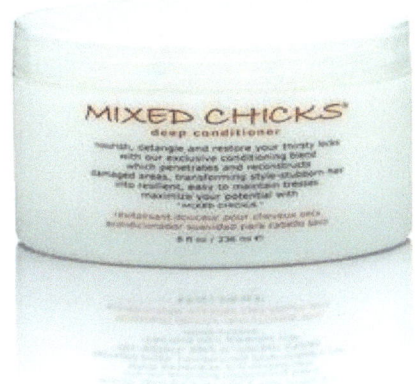

MIXED CHICKS

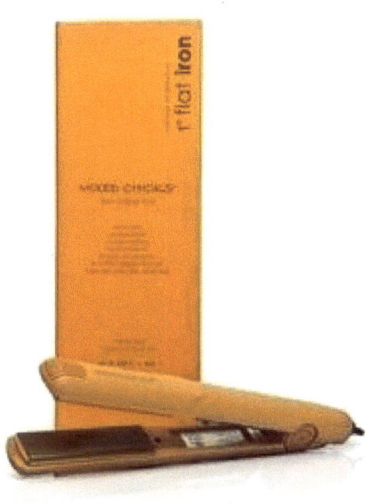

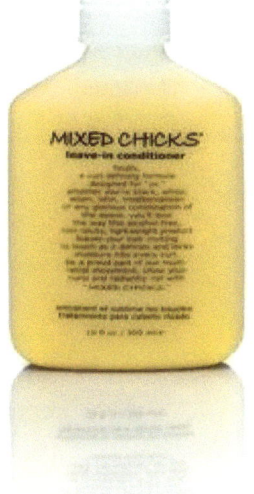

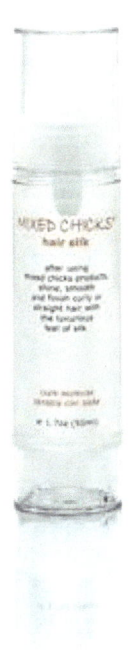

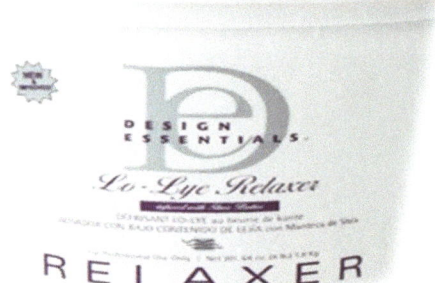

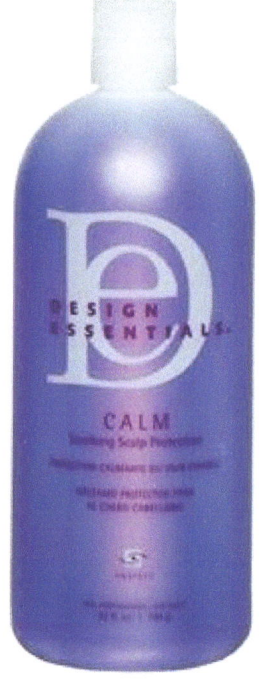

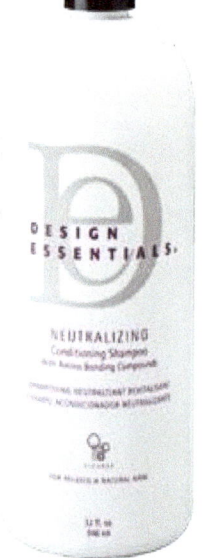

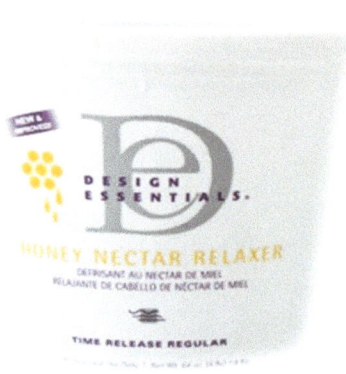